GUT HEALTH FOR BEGINNERS

BOOST ENERGY, BALANCE WEIGHT, AND TRANSFORM YOUR WELLNESS THROUGH THE MICROBIOME

JORDAN ELLIS

Contents

INTRODUCTION

A few years ago, my life was an endless cycle of fatigue, unpredictable digestive issues, and a confusing battle with fluctuating weight. Like many adults, I was caught in the daily grind—juggling work responsibilities, family duties, and a bit of a social life. However, my energy levels were like a stormy sea, and my weight seemed to have a mind of its own. A series of doctor visits followed, each ending with a new prescription, yet none brought me closer to the relief I desperately sought. Amid this whirlwind of frustration and hopelessness, I discovered an unexpected beacon of hope: the fascinating world of the gut microbiome.

To say I was skeptical at first would be an understatement. The idea that many tiny organisms in my gut could unlock the path to better health seemed unbelievable. But as I explored this hidden ecosystem and worked to understand its complexities, I experienced a remarkable transformation. My energy levels not only revived but reached new heights. My digestive system found its rhythm, and a sense of balance I had not felt in years wrapped around me, bringing a profound sense of relief and renewed hope.

This personal journey sparked a strong desire to share the knowledge I had gained, so this book aims to guide you, the beginner, along the path of understanding and optimizing gut health. I want to simplify complex scientific ideas into clear, actionable insights that fit seamlessly into your daily life. Whether you are here due to digestive issues, a quest for greater vitality, or pure curiosity about the gut's overall role in your health, this book is your practical, evidence-based guide. The importance of gut health goes beyond a trend; it is the foundation of holistic wellness, and this book is your reliable companion, always there to support and guide you.

Research shows the gut's crucial role in regulating energy levels, managing weight, and supporting mental health. Did you know that about 70% of your immune system is in your gut or that a healthy gut can reduce anxiety and boost your mood? These insights highlight the deep connection between our bodily systems and the need to prioritize gut health. Writing this book represents the peak of my passion and a personal mission to guide others toward wellness. My goal is to clarify the idea of gut health, breaking the misconception that achieving optimal wellness relies on strict diets or costly supplements. Instead, I promote gradual, informed changes in lifestyle that align with your circumstances, empowering you to take control of your health in a way that suits you best.

In the following chapters, we will explore the complexities of the microbiome and its significant impact on your health. You will learn about dietary changes that promote a healthy gut, lifestyle tweaks worth adopting, and the fascinating gut-brain connection that significantly influences your emotional and psychological well-being. This narrative goes beyond a simple diet guide; it serves as a holistic manifesto for well-being. This book is intended for adults who, regardless of their health knowledge or digestive health condition, are interested in nutrition and wish to improve their quality of life. It is designed for beginners seeking clear and straightforward advice. By the end of the book, I promise you will have the tools to improve your digestion, boost your energy, and enhance your overall health.

I encourage you to embark on this journey with curiosity and openness. Embracing small, sustainable lifestyle changes can catalyze significant, lasting improvements in your health. Together, we will explore how caring for your gut can transform your life. This book's essence is that understanding your gut's complexities marks a significant step toward better health and is designed to be your mentor and partner on this journey. As you read through these pages, you will discover a wealth of information and inspiration to make meaningful changes. Let us begin this path toward wellness, taking one thoughtful step at a time.

CHAPTER 1

UNDERSTANDING THE BASICS

Have you ever wondered how some people seem to exude vitality, seemingly immune to weight fluctuations or digestive problems? This question often crossed my mind, especially during those sluggish afternoons when my energy levels dipped. Surprisingly, the answer may lie within our bodies—in the gut, to be precise. This internal world is teeming with diverse microorganisms, a bustling ecosystem that operates beneath our conscious awareness yet plays a fundamental role in shaping our health.

In this chapter, we will embark on a fascinating, detailed journey into the heart of the microbiome. This microscopic community, although small, wields an extraordinary influence over our health and well-being. By delving into the complexities of this ecosystem, we pave the way toward unlocking the secrets of vibrant health that seem to elude so many. Understanding the microbiome is about recognizing its constituents and appreciating our synbiotic relationship with these tiny inhabitants. This foundational knowledge is essential for anyone aiming to enhance their well-being, offering insights into our gut health's profound impact on our overall vitality.

WHAT IS THE MICROBIOME?

Let us delve deeper into the essence of the microbiome, an invisible yet bustling metropolis within us. This vast community, made up of trillions of microorganisms such as bacteria, viruses, and fungi, primarily resides in our gut. These microorganisms are not just occupants but diligent workers who contribute tirelessly to our health. They play essential roles in breaking down food, absorbing nutrients, and protecting us from harmful pathogens. These processes are vital because, without this microbial assistance, our bodies would encounter significant challenges in extracting the full nutritional value from our diets, impacting our overall efficiency and health.

The importance of diversity within this microbial ecosystem cannot be overstated. Picture your microbiome as a vibrant, thriving ecosystem analogous to a rainforest. In the same way that rich biodiversity sustains a rainforest's health, a varied population of microbes ensures the equilibrium and resilience of your gut. This microbial diversity equips your gut to ward off diseases more effectively, as a broad array of microbes can perform a comprehensive spectrum of functions. They not only combat pathogens but also synthesize crucial vitamins. Conversely, a homogeneous microbial population can leave your gut susceptible to disruptions and illnesses, akin to a city functioning with only one kind of labor force, which would inevitably falter without a diverse set of skills.

The development of our microbiome is a dynamic process shaped by numerous factors from the very beginning of our lives. The mode of our birth sets the initial stage of microbial colonization; infants born through vaginal delivery encounter distinct microbes compared to those born via cesarean section. Babies born vaginally are first colonized by beneficial bacteria from the mother's birth canal and gut, including lactobacillus and bifidobacterium. In contrast, C-section babies initially acquire mainly skin and environmental bacteria like staphylococcus. These differences affect early immune system development and can persist for months or years. However, they may eventually become less distinct, especially with early interventions like vaginal seeding and breastfeeding that can help bridge some of these differences. The latter has a profound impact, offering essential nutrients that promote beneficial bacteria growth.

As we progress through life, our urban or rural surroundings continuously introduce new microbial varieties into our system, enriching the unique microbial tapestry of our gut. This microbial landscape is constantly changing, shaped by our diet, lifestyle, and even the medications we consume. Food can significantly shift the microbial balance, favoring some species while suppressing others. For instance, a fiber-rich diet promotes the flourishing of protective bacteria. Conversely, despite their utility in combating infections, antibiotics can indiscriminately decimate microbial populations, eradicating beneficial microbes alongside harmful ones.

Thankfully, the adaptability of our microbiome offers a beacon of hope. Adopting a diet rich in varied and wholesome foods such as fruits, vegetables, whole grains, and lean proteins and maintaining healthy lifestyles can foster a robust and diverse microbiome that bolsters our health and well-being. Understanding the microbiome concept unveils a powerful ally within us, capable of transforming our health. This microscopic universe is instrumental in optimizing our energy levels, maintaining a healthy weight, and enhancing our digestive efficiency. By cherishing and cultivating our microbiome, we unlock a path to enduring health and vitality, harnessing the full potential of this hidden world to uplift our quality of life significantly.

MEET THE PROBIOTICS: YOUR GUT ALLIES

Again, visualize your digestive system as a bustling metropolis, this time with probiotics as the diligent residents constantly working to uphold your health. These beneficial bacteria, like lactobacillus and bifidobacterium, are pivotal for digestion. They break down fibrous foods into short-chain fatty acids (SCFAs), essential fuel sources for the cells lining your gut. This process is akin to a well-oiled assembly line, where raw materials (fiber) are transformed into vital energy, underscoring the crucial role of probiotics in fostering a balanced and thriving gut ecosystem.

Discovering the sources of these friendly microbes is an adventure into culinary tradition and modern nutrition science.

Naturally occurring in fermented foods, probiotics have been a cornerstone of human diets for millennia. Yogurt, kefir, and sauerkraut are not just culinary delights; they are teeming with life, offering a palatable means of enriching your gut health. The fermentation process of these foods is a natural phenomenon where beneficial bacteria feast on sugars and starches, producing lactic acid. This acts to preserve these foods and promotes the growth of a beneficial microbial community within them. Due to dietary restrictions or preferences, a range of supplements is available for those who find it challenging to incorporate a sufficient variety of probiotic-rich foods into their daily meals. These include capsules, tablets, and powders, providing a convenient alternative to directly consuming fermented foods.

Probiotics do more than aid digestion—they also play a prominent role in mental health and may help alleviate symptoms like irritable bowel syndrome (IBS). This common ailment, characterized by cramping and bloating, can be reduced by enhancing gut health through probiotic intake. Furthermore, recent research indicates that probiotics can improve mood and decrease anxiety, owing to their effect on the gut-brain axis. The gut-brain axis is an intricate communication system that links the gastrointestinal tract to the brain, highlighting the profound connection between our digestive health and mental well-being. This connection is so strong that a healthy gut can positively influence our mental health.

Dispelling myths about probiotics is crucial for understanding their health role. The notion that one probiotic works for everyone is a misconception. Different strains of probiotics serve various purposes, and their effectiveness can differ widely among individuals depending on specific health conditions and needs. Moreover, probiotics offer numerous health benefits but are not a panacea for every issue. Their optimal use occurs when integrated into a health strategy emphasizing a balanced diet and a healthy lifestyle. Relying solely on probiotics without considering other health factors, like diet and exercise, would be akin to expecting a single type of worker to maintain an entire city. Probiotics are a powerful tool for enhancing well-being, but they are most effective when complemented by a holistic approach to overall health.

Reflection Section: Exploring Probiotic Options

Think about your daily routine and consider how integrating probiotics can enhance your well-being. Evaluate your current dietary habits and pinpoint any digestive discomfort or fluctuations in mood you may experience. Natural sources of probiotics, like kefir, yogurt, or sauerkraut, can easily be incorporated into your meals to support gut health. If these fermented foods are new to you, delve into a culinary adventure by trying out recipes that feature these probiotic-rich ingredients.

Probiotic supplements offer a convenient alternative for those with dietary limitations or personal preferences restricting their consumption of such foods. However, when selecting a supplement, it is crucial to identify your specific health objectives. Different probiotic strains enhance health, from digestive function to immune system bolstering. Aim to select a product that aligns with your unique health needs, ensuring that probiotics complement your overall lifestyle and dietary habits.

As we delve deeper into the intricacies of gut health, it becomes clear that probiotics represent a crucial yet singular component of a much larger ecosystem. Their beneficial role within the gut microbiome is undeniable, supporting a healthy digestive system and contributing to our overall health. However, the effectiveness of probiotics is significantly enhanced when part of a holistic health strategy, which incorporates a diverse, nutrient-rich diet, consistent physical activity, and proper hydration. Incorporating a daily serving of fermented foods or a probiotic supplement tailored to your health requirements is a proactive step toward nurturing and maintaining a balanced gut microbiome. By doing so, you not only support your digestive health but also contribute to your body's resilience and vitality, reinforcing the foundation for a thriving inner ecosystem.

PREBIOTICS: FEEDING YOUR FRIENDLY FLORA

Similarly to my other metaphors, imagine your gut as a thriving neighborhood bustling with life and activity. Just like any community, it needs proper nutrition to flourish. This is where prebiotics come into play. Prebiotics are non-digestible fibers, unlike probiotics, which are live bacteria. They serve as food for these beneficial bacteria. They help nourish and promote the growth of good bacteria in your gut, creating a balanced environment. Think of prebiotics as the fertilizer that enriches your garden, ensuring your plants grow strong and healthy. Inulin and fructooligosaccharides (FOS) are two common prebiotics that play a crucial role in maintaining this balance, and these prebiotics support a balanced gut microbiome by encouraging the proliferation of helpful bacteria essential for overall health and well-being.

You might wonder where to find these beneficial prebiotics in your daily diet. Many of them hide in plain sight, in foods you might already enjoy. Garlic, onions, and leeks are some of the best sources. They add flavor to your meals and also feed your gut flora. Bananas, especially when they are slightly green, are another excellent source. They make for a convenient snack or a delicious addition to smoothies. Whole grains like barley and oats and legumes like lentils and chickpeas are also rich in prebiotics. Incorporating these foods into your diet is a simple way to nurture your gut and support your overall health.

The magic happens when prebiotics and probiotics join forces. This combination is known as "synbiotics." When you consume both, prebiotics feed the probiotics, enhancing their ability to thrive in your gut. It is like providing the perfect fuel for your body's internal engine. This synergy can be found in certain foods and supplements designed to maximize gut health. For example, a bowl of yogurt topped with sliced bananas and a sprinkle of oats is delicious and a potent synbiotic meal. Integrating synbiotic foods into your diet can optimize your gut environment, allowing beneficial bacteria to flourish and support your health in countless ways.

The benefits of prebiotics extend beyond just nurturing your gut flora. They significantly improve gut barrier function, which is the gut's ability to act as a protective shield between your internal environment and the outside world. A strong gut barrier helps prevent unwanted substances from entering your bloodstream, reducing inflammation and disease risk. Prebiotics also enhance mineral absorption, particularly calcium and magnesium, vital for bone health and numerous bodily functions. By strengthening the gut lining, prebiotics contribute to a more robust immune system, better digestion, and overall vitality. Embracing prebiotics in your diet is a step toward bolstering your health from the inside out.

Incorporating prebiotics into your daily routine does not have to be complicated. Start by adding more garlic and onions to your cooking. Experiment with whole grains and legumes in your meals. Consider starting your day with a banana or enjoying a bowl of oatmeal for breakfast. These small changes can make a substantial impact on your gut health. As you explore the world of prebiotics, you will find that nourishing your gut is beneficial and deliciously satisfying. Embrace the power of prebiotics and watch as your health flourishes, one fiber-rich bite at a time.

THE GUT-BRAIN AXIS: A TWO-WAY STREET

Imagine your gut and brain as two best friends who constantly chat and share secrets. This communication is the gut-brain axis, a fascinating concept highlighting the ongoing dialogue between these two organs. The gut and brain continually converse, linked by a complex network of hormones, chemicals, and nerves. The vagus nerve is the main highway for this communication, transmitting signals back and forth. This connection is not just about sending messages; it is vital in regulating mood, cognitive function, and overall mental health. When your gut feels good, your mind follows suit, and vice versa. Understanding this connection can help us see why a healthy gut promotes a healthy mind.

The gut impacts mental health in several profound ways. One of the most intriguing aspects is its role in producing neurotransmitters. For example, serotonin, often called the "feel-good hormone," is primarily produced in the gut. This neurotransmitter influences mood, sleep, and even appetite. A well-balanced gut promotes serotonin production, helping to improve mood and ease anxiety or depression. The gut microbiota —a diverse community of bacteria in the digestive system—also plays a crucial role in managing stress. When disrupted by stress, this delicate balance shifts, affecting how the body responds to anxiety and tension. Maintaining gut health can help stabilize your emotions and improve your mental well-being.

On the other hand, mental health can significantly impact your gut. Stress and emotions are not just fleeting feelings; they can have tangible effects on your digestive system. Stress often triggers gut motility and secretion changes, sometimes resulting in gastrointestinal issues like constipation or diarrhea. This can lead to functional gut disorders, where stress exacerbates symptoms and creates a cycle of discomfort. Psychological aspects like depression and anxiety can also influence gut health, making it crucial to address both mental and physical aspects of well-being. Recognizing the gut-brain axis means acknowledging the power of emotions over digestion and vice versa.

Supporting the gut-brain connection involves a few practical strategies. Mindfulness and meditation can be potent practices in this area. These practices encourage relaxation and stress reduction, supporting a healthy gut environment. (We will explore this more deeply in Chapter 8: Understanding and Managing Stress for Digestive Health.) Setting aside a few minutes each day for mindfulness can calm your mind and, in turn, your gut. Incorporating diets rich in omega-3 fatty acids in foods like salmon, walnuts, and flaxseeds is also beneficial. Omega-3s support brain health and can enhance communication between the gut and brain, promoting a balanced mood and reducing inflammation. By making these lifestyle changes, you can nurture the connection between your stomach and brain, improving mental and physical health.

Understanding the gut-brain axis provides a holistic approach to health that accounts for the interconnectedness of our body's systems. Caring for your gut supports your mental health, creating a cycle of wellness that benefits both body and mind. This bidirectional relationship reminds us that our bodies are complex and deeply interconnected, and small changes can ripple through our entire being. Embracing this perspective empowers us to take charge of our health, knowing that our choices can have far-reaching effects on how we feel daily.

GUT HEALTH AND IMMUNITY: THE FIRST LINE OF DEFENSE

Picture your gut as a bustling defense headquarters for your body, where the immune system gears up to protect you from invaders. The gut plays a noteworthy role in your immune system function. It houses a crucial component known as the gut-associated lymphoid tissue (GALT), a surveillance system that constantly monitors and responds to potential threats. GALT works closely with the gut microbiota, the community of microorganisms in your digestive tract, to maintain a harmonious balance. These microorganisms interact with immune cells, training them to distinguish between harmful invaders and harmless substances. This interaction is fundamental because it helps the immune system efficiently target pathogens while avoiding unnecessary inflammation. A healthy gut is like a well-oiled engine, ensuring that your body's defenses are always ready to act when needed.

A well-balanced gut microbiome serves as a formidable shield against disease. When your gut is healthy, it prevents the overgrowth of pathogenic bacteria that may lead to infections. By maintaining a diverse and balanced microbial environment, your gut microbiome can outcompete harmful bacteria, reducing their chances of taking hold. Furthermore, the gut's influence on inflammatory pathways is profound. Inflammation, when unchecked, can contribute to a host of chronic diseases. A healthy gut helps modulate these pathways, reducing chronic inflammation and promoting overall health. This protective effect underscores the importance of nurturing your gut to prevent acute infections and long-term health issues.

Consider incorporating various immune-boosting foods into your diet to bolster your gut and immune health. Fermented foods like kimchi and miso are delicious and rich in probiotics that support gut flora. Leafy greens like kale and spinach provide vital nutrients and antioxidants, strengthening your body's defenses. Packed with vitamin C and other antioxidants, berries offer a tasty way to enhance immunity. Also, zinc-rich foods, such as nuts and seeds, are essential in sustaining a robust immune system. You can naturally support your gut and fortify your immune defenses by including these foods in your daily meals.

In addition to diet, lifestyle habits play a pivotal role in boosting gut immunity. Routine physical activity is one of the best ways to enhance gut health and immune function. Exercise promotes circulation, reduces stress, and supports a healthy weight, all contributing to a resilient immune system. Adequate sleep is equally important. While you rest, your body repairs and rejuvenates, allowing the immune system to function optimally. Managing stress is another crucial factor. Chronic stress can diminish the immune system and disrupt gut health. Introducing stress-reducing practices, like meditation or yoga, can help maintain balance and support your body's defenses. By adopting these habits, you create a lifestyle that nurtures your gut and strengthens your immune system.

As we wrap up our exploration of the gut's role in immunity, remember that your gut is not just a digestive organ but a vital part of your overall health. Understanding its influence on the immune system enables you to make informed choices that enhance your well-being. Whether through diet, exercise, or stress management, every positive change contributes to a healthier, more resilient you. Embrace these practices, and let your gut be your guide to a vibrant and fortified life.

CHAPTER 2

THE SCIENCE OF GUT HEALTH

As I sit here enjoying my morning coffee, I am reminded of the profound importance of gut flora diversity. This concept first struck me during a brunch with a friend fresh from the Amazon. Her vivid descriptions of the diverse ecosystems she encountered, each teeming with a rich variety of plant and animal life, drew a striking parallel to our guts—miniature rainforests bustling with different species of bacteria, each with a unique role in maintaining the health of this ecosystem. Just as biodiversity is crucial for the stability and resilience of natural environments, a diverse gut flora is equally vital for our health.

AN INTRODUCTION TO GUT DIVERSITY

Like a team of superheroes, your gut is always ready to face any challenge. Each type of bacteria brings unique skills, from breaking down complex carbohydrates to modulating immune responses. This diversity is a defense against pathogenic invasions, much like how many plant and animal species protect a rainforest from disease. When an ecosystem is diverse, it can bounce back more quickly from disruptions. Your gut works in the same way; a multitude of microbial players fortify its resilience against diseases and infections. This adaptability and resilience of your gut microbiome should reassure you about your body's ability to handle challenges.

However, as discussed in the previous chapter, many factors influence your gut flora's diversity. Diet is a major player here. Consider the stark contrast between a Western diet, lacking fiber and rich in processed foods, and a traditional diet rich in whole, plant-based foods. The former often leads to a less diverse microbiome, increasing the risk of health issues. Meanwhile, a diet abundant in fruits, vegetables, and whole grains fosters a robust microbial community. Our environment also plays a role. Those living in rural areas often have more diverse gut microbiota than urban dwellers, possibly due to greater exposure to varied natural microbes. Again, lifestyle choices, like the use of antibiotics, can also impact microbial diversity. Other lifestyle choices we have touched on that impact gut health include stress, exercise, and sleep patterns. For instance, chronic stress can disrupt the balance of bacteria in your gut, while regular exercise can promote a diverse gut microbiome. While antibiotics are sometimes necessary, they can reduce the variety of bacteria in your gut, underscoring the importance of using them judiciously.

The benefits of a diverse gut flora are extensive. It enhances metabolic functions, helping your body efficiently break down complex carbohydrates into usable energy. This process is essential for maintaining steady energy levels and preventing weight gain. Additionally, a diverse microbiome supports your immune system, fine-tuning its ability to respond to threats without overreacting and causing inflammation. This is essential for preventing chronic diseases such as obesity, diabetes, and even some neurological disorders. Maintaining various gut bacteria creates a resilient internal environment that supports physical and mental health.

So, how can you boost the diversity in your gut? One effective strategy is incorporating more fermented foods like yogurt, kimchi, or kombucha into your diet. These foods are natural sources of probiotics, introducing beneficial bacteria into your gut and enriching its microbial community. For instance, you can begin your day with a bowl of fresh fruit and yogurt, have a side of kimchi with your lunch, or enjoy a glass of kombucha as a midday refreshment. Fermented foods have undergone lacto-fermentation, where natural bacteria feed on the food's starch and sugar, creating lactic acid. This preserves the food and produces beneficial enzymes, B vitamins, omega-3 fatty acids, and probiotic strains. Another approach is to vary the plant-based foods you consume. Regularly changing the fruits, vegetables, and grains you eat provides a range of fibers and nutrients that different bacteria thrive on. This dietary variety is akin to planting a diverse garden, ensuring your gut flora has everything it needs to flourish.

Reflection Section: Cultivating a Diverse Gut

Reflect deeply on your current dietary practices and the environment around you. Consider making simple yet effective adjustments to enhance the diversity of your diet, which could dramatically increase the variety of beneficial microbes in your gut. Imagine the potential benefits of introducing a new vegetable to your plate each week or experimenting with a fermented delicacy you have previously bypassed. These seemingly minor dietary modifications could pave the way for significant improvements in your gut health, ultimately elevating your overall well-being. The benefits of maintaining a diverse microbiome should motivate you to change your diet positively.

As you embark on this journey, observing the changes that unfold meticulously is crucial. These could range from improved digestion and nutrient absorption to a noticeable uplift in energy and mood. To capture the full spectrum of these transformations, maintaining a comprehensive food diary during this exploration phase could prove invaluable. In this diary, record the foods you consume and any shifts in your physical sensations and emotional states. This detailed tracking will enable you to identify patterns and correlations between your dietary choices and their impacts on your gut health. Embrace the understanding that nurturing a diverse microbiome extends beyond a singular action—it is a continuous exploration marked by patience, curiosity, and a readiness to evolve your dietary habits. By committing to this path, you will uncover that enriching your gut flora is not merely an act of self-care but an enriching journey that fosters a more vibrant, resilient, and healthful life.

THE ROLE OF FIBER IN DIGESTIVE HEALTH

Fiber often gets a reputation for being the dull part of nutrition, but it is a powerhouse for your gut health. If your digestive system is a well-oiled machine, fiber is the lubricant that keeps it running smoothly. Two main types of dietary fiber play distinct roles in maintaining digestive health: soluble and insoluble. Soluble fiber in foods like oats and beans dissolves in water to make a gel-like substance. This type of fiber slows digestion, helping your body absorb nutrients effectively. It is also essential in lowering cholesterol and regulating blood sugar levels. On the other hand, insoluble fiber, found in whole grains and vegetables, does not dissolve in water. Instead, it adds mass to stool and helps food go more quickly through the stomach and intestines. This is essential for preventing constipation and keeping the digestive tract clean.

When you consume fiber, you are not just feeding yourself— you are feeding the beneficial bacteria in your gut. Soluble fiber undergoes fermentation in the colon, where these bacteria convert it into short-chain fatty acids. These SCFAs fuel your gut cells, promoting a healthy gut lining and reducing inflammation. They have also been shown to play a role in regulating appetite and body weight. Meanwhile, insoluble fiber contributes to stool bulk, which, again, aids in maintaining regular bowel movements. Regularity is more than just a matter of comfort; it is a sign of a healthy digestive system. By ensuring that waste moves efficiently through your intestines, fiber helps reduce the risk of developing digestive disorders like diverticulosis and hemorrhoids.

The benefits of fiber go beyond aiding digestion; it plays a protective role against several severe health conditions. Research has consistently shown that high fiber intake reduces the risk of developing colorectal cancer. This protective effect results from fiber's ability to accelerate food movement through the digestive system, minimizing the time harmful substances remain in contact with the intestinal lining. Additionally, fiber helps lower the risk of cardiovascular disease by lowering cholesterol levels and improving blood pressure. Epidemiological studies have shown that populations with high-fiber diets tend to have lower incidences of heart disease. These protective effects highlight the importance of making fiber a staple in your diet.

Incorporating more fiber into your meals might seem daunting, but a few simple adjustments can become a natural part of your routine. Start by gradually increasing your intake of fiber-rich foods. This approach adjusts your digestive system and helps prevent bloating and discomfort. Begin your day with a bowl of oatmeal topped with fresh fruits for a fiber boost. Swap out white bread for whole-grain options, and consider adding beans or lentils to your salads or soups. Another key to optimizing fiber's benefits is staying hydrated. Water helps fiber do its job by ensuring it moves smoothly through your digestive tract. Try drinking eight glasses of water daily, but this is not a set amount. Adjust based on your activity and climate.

Making these small but impactful changes can significantly enhance your digestive health. As you introduce more fiber into your diet, you will probably notice improvements in how you feel daily. The benefits, from better digestion to increased energy levels, are worth the effort. Plus, by prioritizing fiber, you are not just improving your gut health but investing in your long-term well-being.

UNDERSTANDING LEAKY GUT: CAUSES AND EFFECTS

Imagine your gut as a sturdy wall, selectively letting beneficial nutrients pass through while keeping harmful substances out. The "leaky gut" concept challenges this image, suggesting that the wall has developed tiny holes or cracks. This increased intestinal permeability can allow partially digested food particles, toxins, and microbes to escape into the bloodstream, potentially triggering inflammation and other health issues. The tight passages in the intestinal lining are at the heart of this issue. These are supposed to act as gatekeepers. When these junctions weaken, they can no longer effectively control what passes through, potentially leading to various health problems. Some researchers believe this permeability may be linked to autoimmune diseases, when the body mistakenly attacks its tissues, viewing them as foreign invaders. Though more research is needed, understanding this concept emphasizes the significance of preserving a healthy gut lining.

Several factors contribute to the development of a leaky gut.

Diet is a significant one. Ingesting high amounts of sugar and processed foods can irritate the gut lining, exacerbating permeability issues. These foods often have additives and preservatives that may disrupt the balance of gut bacteria, further weakening the intestinal wall. Chronic stress is another culprit. Your body releases hormones that can harm gut health when stressed. This physiological response can lead to inflammation, making the gut lining more susceptible to leaks. It is not just the occasional stressful day that poses a risk but prolonged periods of stress that can impact gut integrity. These lifestyle influences underscore the importance of mindful eating and stress management in preserving gut health (we explore this more in Chapter 4: Building Gut-Friendly Habits).

The symptoms and conditions associated with leaky gut can differ significantly, making it a bit of a mystery for many. Digestive discomfort is a common complaint, with symptoms like bloating, gas, and food sensitivities often reported. Beyond the gut, a leaky gut may manifest as skin issues such as eczema or acne, suggesting a link between intestinal health and skin clarity. Some people also experience fatigue, which can be chronic and debilitating, pointing to a possible connection between leaky gut and chronic fatigue syndrome. Though these symptoms can be vague and overlap with other conditions, they highlight the potential wide-reaching effects of a compromised gut barrier.

Addressing a leaky gut involves supporting and restoring the integrity of the gut lining. Adopting an anti-inflammatory diet is a powerful starting point. Such a diet focuses on whole, unprocessed foods with antioxidants and omega-3 fatty acids that aid lower inflammation and support gut health. Incorporating foods like leafy greens, berries, and fatty fish into your meals can provide the nutrients needed to nourish your gut. Supplements like L-glutamine and zinc also play a role in gut repair. L-glutamine is an amino acid. It helps maintain the intestinal barrier and supports cell regeneration. Meanwhile, zinc is known for its role in immune function and can aid in healing the gut lining. By combining these dietary and supplementary strategies, you can work toward strengthening your gut and improving overall health.

Although incorporating these changes may seem daunting initially, beginning small can lead to significant improvements. Begin by gradually introducing anti-inflammatory foods into your daily meals, and consider consulting a healthcare professional for personalized supplement recommendations. Again, using a journal to track your symptoms and dietary changes can help you pinpoint what works best for your body. As you make these adjustments, you may notice reduced digestive discomfort and improved overall well-being. These steps address leaky gut and create a foundation for better health, empowering you to take control of your wellness.

THE IMPACT OF GUT HEALTH ON MOOD AND COGNITION

Have you ever observed how your mood can shift after a hearty meal or how stress can upset your stomach? This is no mere coincidence. The gut produces neurotransmitters, the chemical messengers that influence mood and cognition. Serotonin, often dubbed the "happiness hormone," is produced mainly in the gut.

This neurotransmitter is crucial for regulating mood, sleep, and even appetite. However, serotonin does not work alone. Gut bacteria also influence dopamine pathways, which affect pleasure and motivation. The gut is like a bustling factory, where these critical chemicals are manufactured and released, impacting how we feel and think.

The connection between mental well-being and gut health is not just speculative. Research has shown significant connections between the two, particularly in mental health disorders like depression and anxiety. Studies have highlighted how gut dysbiosis, an imbalance of gut bacteria, can correlate with increased anxiety levels. Changes in gut microbiota can disrupt the production of neurotransmitters, leading to mood swings and emotional instability. Probiotic interventions have been studied for their potential to alleviate symptoms of mood disorders. By restoring balance in the gut, probiotics can improve mood and reduce anxiety, showcasing the profound influence of gut health on mental states.

Supporting mental well-being through gut health is not abstract; you can actively work on it. Start by incorporating omega-3-rich foods like salmon, walnuts, and flaxseeds. These foods support brain health and enhance the production of neurotransmitters. Again, mindfulness practices can also help reduce stress, benefiting your gut and mind. Deep breathing or meditation can calm your nervous system, reducing stress-induced gut disturbances. Adding these practices to your everyday routine can nurture a healthier connection between your gut and brain, improving mental health.

Real-life stories often bring these concepts to life. Take Zola, for example, who struggled with anxiety and digestive issues for years. After learning about the gut-brain connection, she started incorporating probiotics and omega-3s into her diet and practiced mindfulness regularly. Over time, she noticed a significant improvement in her mood and a reduction in anxiety symptoms. Zola's experience highlights how small, intentional changes can lead to meaningful improvements in mental health. Her story is just one of many that illustrate the powerful impact of caring for your gut to enhance your overall well-being.

These insights into the gut-brain connection underscore the importance of holistic health. By understanding how intertwined our bodies are, we can make informed decisions that benefit our mental and physical well-being, building a foundation for a more balanced and fulfilling life.

INFLAMMATION AND THE GUT: THE HIDDEN CONNECTION

As you go about your day, it might not cross your mind that your gut and inflammation could be conversing. The correlation between gut health and systemic inflammation is significant, affecting how your body responds to various challenges. As mentioned, your gut lining acts like a defensive barrier, selectively allowing nutrients to pass through while keeping harmful invaders out. When that barrier becomes compromised, often described as increased gut permeability, it can cascade inflammatory responses throughout your body. This is where your gut microbiota comes into play. These microorganisms help regulate inflammation by interacting with your immune system, teaching it to respond appropriately without overreacting. A balanced gut can help keep inflammation in check, preventing it from spiraling out of control and affecting overall health.

Chronic inflammation is a sneaky contributor to many health issues. It is like a slow-burning fire that can cause damage over time. Persistent inflammation has been connected to multiple chronic illnesses. This includes diseases like metabolic syndrome and type 2 diabetes. When inflammation becomes a constant presence, it disrupts normal bodily functions, affecting how you metabolize sugars and fats. This can lead to other metabolic disorders like insulin resistance, a precursor to diabetes. The role of inflammation in chronic diseases underscores the importance of maintaining a healthy gut. Maintaining inflammation reduces your risk of developing these conditions and supports a healthier you.

Your diet plays a crucial role in either fueling or fighting inflammation. Specific dietary patterns can exacerbate inflammation, leading to health problems. Diets with lots of processed foods and trans fats are particularly detrimental. These foods often have additives and preservatives that can irritate your gut lining, further promoting inflammation. Conversely, adopting an anti-inflammatory diet rich in antioxidants can significantly help. Foods like berries, leafy greens, and nuts contain these potent compounds, which help neutralize free radicals and reduce inflammation. Embracing an anti-inflammatory diet is like giving your body a toolkit to combat the fire of inflammation, supporting both your gut and overall health.

To reduce inflammation through gut health, consider making some lifestyle changes. One effective strategy is following a Mediterranean diet, emphasizing whole grains, fruits, vegetables, lean proteins, and healthy fats. This diet is renowned for its anti-inflammatory properties and correlates with a lower risk of chronic diseases. Also, adding regular physical activity into your routine is essential. Exercise helps reduce inflammation by improving circulation and promoting the release of anti-inflammatory substances. Whether it is a brisk walk, yoga, or a workout at the gym, staying active is a simple yet powerful way to support your gut and reduce inflammation. These changes do not have to happen overnight but can be gradually integrated into your life for lasting benefits.

Now that we have explored the intricate ties between gut health and inflammation, it is clear how integral your gut is to maintaining overall wellness. Understanding and addressing inflammation can enhance your health from the inside out.

THE CONNECTION BETWEEN GUT HEALTH AND SLEEP: UNLOCKING RESTFUL NIGHTS

As discussed, your gut is home to trillions of microorganisms that form an intricate ecosystem known as the gut microbiota. These microorganisms do not just digest food; they also communicate with your body's circadian rhythm—the internal clock that regulates your sleep-wake cycle.

Gut Microbiota and Circadian Rhythms

Research shows that disrupted gut microbiota can disturb your circadian rhythm, meaning poor sleep quality and irregular sleep patterns. For instance, an imbalance in gut bacteria, often caused by eating lots of processed foods or stress, can produce inflammatory compounds that interfere with your body's ability to regulate sleep. This imbalance may also affect the production of neurotransmitters and hormones essential for a good night's sleep.

The Role of Serotonin and Melatonin

Serotonin, often called the "happiness hormone," is vital for mood regulation and serves as a precursor to melatonin, the hormone that governs your sleep cycle. About 90% of your body's serotonin is produced in the gut. When your gut is healthy and functioning optimally, serotonin levels are sufficient to ensure that your body can produce adequate melatonin, helping you fall asleep more quickly and stay asleep longer. Conversely, poor diet, stress, or illness can decrease serotonin production when gut health deteriorates. This reduction affects melatonin levels, potentially causing insomnia, restless sleep, or difficulty maintaining a regular sleep schedule. This link underscores the importance of maintaining a balanced gut for consistent, high-quality sleep.

Practical Tips for Gut-Supportive Sleep

As we have seen already, improving your gut health does not

have to be complicated. Simple dietary and lifestyle changes can significantly enhance sleep quality by nurturing a thriving microbiota. Here are some actionable tips:

1. **Add Tryptophan-Rich Foods**: Tryptophan is an amino acid that your body uses to produce serotonin. Foods like oats, bananas, nuts, seeds, turkey, and eggs are excellent sources of tryptophan. Including these in your evening meal can support serotonin production and, by extension, melatonin synthesis

2. **Incorporate Prebiotics and Probiotics**: Prebiotics, such as those found in garlic, onions, and asparagus, feed the beneficial bacteria in your gut. Conversely, probiotics are found in yogurt, kefir, and fermented foods like kimchi. Together, they can help maintain a healthy microbial balance that supports digestion and sleep.

3. **Limit Late-Night Eating**. Eating late can disrupt your gut's natural rhythms, which are closely tied to your body's circadian clock. Try to finish your last meal at least two to three hours before bedtime to give your digestive system a chance to rest.

4. **Stay Hydrated**: Dehydration can negatively impact gut function and, in turn, your sleep quality. Ensure you drink enough water throughout the day, but avoid excessive liquids before bed to prevent nighttime awakenings.

5. **Manage Stress**: Chronic stress can damage gut health, disrupting its ability to produce the hormones and neurotransmitters needed for restful sleep. Incorporate stress-reducing practices like mindfulness, yoga, or deep breathing exercises into your daily routine.

Consider the story of Emily, a busy professional who struggled with sleepless nights and groggy mornings. Emily made a few changes after learning about the connection between her gut health and sleep. She added a small bowl of yogurt with bananas and a handful of almonds to her evening routine, providing her body with probiotics and tryptophan. She also made it a point to avoid late-night snacks and started practicing mindfulness for ten minutes before bed. Within a few weeks, Emily noticed a significant improvement in her sleep quality. She fell asleep faster, stayed asleep longer, and woke up feeling refreshed. Emily's story highlights how small, consistent changes can profoundly affect gut health and sleep quality.

ENVIRONMENTAL FACTORS AND GUT HEALTH

As briefly mentioned, gut health is not isolated but intimately connected to the outside world. Environmental factors significantly shape your microbiome, influencing everything from bacterial diversity to digestive function. Understanding how environmental conditions affect gut health allows you to adapt your dietary and lifestyle choices. This dynamic relationship between your internal ecosystem and external environment requires attention and adaptation throughout the year and across different geographical locations.

Seasonal Changes

As nature cycles through seasons, your gut microbiome undergoes seasonal variations in response to changing food availability, daylight hours, and temperature patterns. Traditional human societies historically experienced significant seasonal shifts in their diets, leading to cyclical changes in their gut bacteria composition. Modern life may have smoothed out some variations, but your body still responds to seasonal cues, affecting appetite, metabolism, and digestive patterns.

Many people experience changes in their eating habits and digestion during winter. Shorter days can affect circadian rhythm, altering gut motility and enzyme production. The natural tendency toward heartier, warming foods during cold weather influences your microbiome composition. Similarly, summer's abundance of fresh fruits and vegetables provides different fiber and nutrients, promoting the growth of seasonal-specific bacterial populations. Understanding these natural rhythms helps you work with, rather than against, your body's seasonal adaptations.

Travel and Gut Adaptation

Traveling across time zones and geographical regions presents unique challenges to your digestive system. The term "traveler's gut" encompasses more than just exposure to unfamiliar bacteria—

it includes changes in meal timing, food choices, water composition, and stress levels. Your microbiome requires time to adapt to new environmental conditions, which explains why digestive issues often accompany travel, even to destinations with high food safety standards.

Altitude changes, different climates, and varying levels of air pollution can all impact your gut function during travel. High-altitude environments may affect digestion due to changes in atmospheric pressure and oxygen levels. Similarly, moving between humid and dry climates can affect your hydration status and, consequently, your digestive function. Preparing your gut for travel through targeted probiotic supplementation and maintaining consistent eating patterns can help ease these transitions.

Environmental Toxins

Modern environments expose the gut to unprecedented chemical compounds that can disrupt microbiome balance. From household cleaning products to agricultural pesticides, these substances can affect the composition and function of gut bacteria. Microplastics, now ubiquitous in our environment, have emerged as a concern for gut health, potentially influencing bacterial communities and intestinal barrier function.

Water quality is vital in this equation, and chlorine and other purification chemicals can affect gut bacteria. While these treatments are necessary for public health, they may have unintended consequences for your microbiome. Air pollution, including indoor air quality, can also impact gut health through the gut-lung axis, highlighting the interconnected nature of environmental exposure and digestive wellness.

Climate Impact on Microbiome

Climate conditions directly influence the bacterial communities living within and around us. Temperature and humidity levels affect the external microbes we encounter and how our bodies regulate internal processes. Research suggests that people in different climate zones harbor distinct microbiome patterns, reflecting long-term environmental adaptation. As global climate patterns shift, these relationships may face new challenges, requiring increased attention to maintaining microbiome resilience.

Extreme weather events and changing seasonal patterns can affect food availability and quality, indirectly impacting gut health through dietary changes. Heat waves may alter food storage needs and increase the risk of foodborne illness, while changing precipitation patterns can affect the nutrient content of soil and, subsequently, our food. Understanding these broader environmental influences helps inform strategies for maintaining gut health in a changing climate.

The link between environmental factors and gut health emphasizes the importance of adaptive strategies. This might include adjusting your diet and supplement routine seasonally, taking extra precautions during travel, and minimizing exposure to environmental toxins where possible. Maintaining awareness of how environmental changes affect your digestion allows you to implement protective measures proactively rather than reactively.

Supporting your gut through environmental challenges requires a combination of protective strategies and adaptive responses. These include filtering your water, choosing organic produce when possible, and adjusting your diet, lifestyle, and habits according to seasonal changes. Consistently practicing healthy habits helps create a resilient gut ecosystem that buffers against environmental stressors while maintaining optimal digestive function regardless of external conditions. The next chapter will explore how recognizing signs of an unhealthy gut is one of the first steps toward transformative health changes.

CHAPTER 3

RECOGNIZING THE SIGNS OF AN UNHEALTHY GUT

Picture yourself at a vibrant dinner gathering encircled by the warmth of friends, savoring a sumptuous meal. Suddenly, an all-too-familiar and unwelcome sensation of bloating strikes. Your abdomen feels uncomfortably tight, as if inflated, making your clothing feel constricting and small. Though often brushed off as a minor nuisance, this discomfort may be your body's method of signaling deeper issues within your gut. Both bloating and gas, while everyday experiences for many, can serve as key indicators of underlying digestive challenges that warrant closer examination. Delving into the origins of these symptoms marks the initial step toward their resolution and enhancing your gut health.

ORIGINS OF BLOATING AND GAS

Understanding the origins of bloating and gas is crucial in taking charge of your gut health. These discomforts often stem from the fermentation process of undigested food within the colon. While integral to digestion, this process can lead to pain and bloating when it intensifies. Food intolerances, such as lactose or fructose, are another common cause. These intolerances emerge when the body struggles to digest certain sugars, leading to gas and bloating. Moreover, small intestinal bacterial overgrowth (SIBO) significantly contributes to these discomforting symptoms. SIBO involves an abnormal proliferation of bacteria within the small intestine. This leads to bloating, diarrhea, and a spectrum of digestive disturbances. Understanding these triggers allows you to implement practical strategies to control your symptoms and enhance your gut health.

SIBO often coexists with conditions like IBS and demands meticulous management to mitigate its symptoms. Identifying bloating and gas triggers is pivotal for effective management. Foods high in FODMAPs (fermentable oligosaccharides, disaccharides, monosaccharides, and polyols)—a group of carbohydrates known for poor absorption in the small intestine— frequently exacerbate bloating for numerous people. Examples of high-FODMAP foods include onions, garlic, beans, and wheat. By minimizing or altogether avoiding these foods, relief from symptoms may be found.

Additionally, eating behaviors significantly influence digestive comfort. Hastily consuming food or eating while distracted can lead to the inadvertent swallowing of air, amplifying gas production. This realization can be enlightening, prompting you to adopt a more mindful approach to eating—slowing down, thoroughly chewing, and fully engaging with the meal. By doing so, you can substantially mitigate bloating and enhance digestive processes. This mindful aspect of eating can help you feel more connected to your body and its needs. Although experiencing bloating and gas occasionally falls within the typical spectrum, persistent symptoms may herald a more severe underlying condition necessitating medical consultation.

If dietary adjustments fail to alleviate discomfort or symptoms are accompanied by unexplained weight loss or blood in the stool, it is crucial to seek professional healthcare guidance. Such manifestations could point toward more intricate digestive disorders that require a thorough evaluation and tailored treatment strategy.

The management of bloating and gas typically involves a blend of lifestyle and dietary modifications. Herbal remedies, such as peppermint tea, offer a natural means of soothing digestive discomfort. Peppermint is endowed with compounds that relax the digestive tract, easing bloating and gas. Once again, including probiotics, especially strains renowned for gas reduction, also proves advantageous. These gas-reducing probiotics can be found in various fermented foods:

- **Lactobacillus Rhamnosus GG**: Present in many yogurts and fermented milk products.

- **Bifidobacterium Longum and Lactis**: Abundant in kefir and aged cheeses.
- **Lactobacillus Plantarum**: Commonly found in sauerkraut, kimchi, and other fermented vegetables.
- **Saccharomyces Boulardii**: A beneficial yeast that occurs naturally in lychee and mangosteen fruits, though it is more commonly taken as a supplement.

Regularly consuming these fermented foods can help maintain healthy gut flora and reduce excessive gas production. These live microorganisms foster a harmonious balance within the gut microbiome, potentially diminishing symptoms. Enveloping these strategies into our daily routine can be critical in effectively managing bloating and gas, ultimately improving overall gut health.

Reflection Section: Identifying Personal Triggers

Take a moment to reflect on your experiences with bloating and gas. These sensations can often serve as your body's way of communicating its need for dietary adjustments or lifestyle changes. I recommend maintaining a detailed food diary for at least one week to better understand your gut's reactions. In this diary, meticulously record everything you consume, including meals, snacks, beverages, and even seemingly minor ingredients. This process of self-discovery can be empowering, as it puts you in control of your gut health and instills confidence in your ability to manage it.

Equally important is to note the timing of your meals and any symptoms you experience afterward, such as bloating, gas, or discomfort. As you compile this diary, pay special attention to how your body responds to different types of meals:

- Do certain foods seem to trigger symptoms consistently?
- Are your symptoms more pronounced at specific times of the day?

This mindful observation can reveal patterns and help you identify potential dietary triggers. For instance, some individuals experience bloating and gas from high-FODMAP foods like onions, garlic, apples, and wheat.

Once you have gathered enough data, experiment with modifying your diet. Start by gradually reducing or eliminating foods you suspect may contribute to discomfort. Common culprits often include dairy products, high-FODMAP foods, and overly processed items. As you adjust your intake of these foods, continue to document any changes in your symptoms. This process of elimination and observation involves removing a suspected trigger food from your diet for a few days and then reintroducing it to see if your symptoms return. If they do, food is likely a trigger for you. This process can enlighten, offering insights into how specific foods impact your gut health.

Additionally, consider the role of eating habits in your digestive well-being. Eating too quickly, consuming meals while distracted, or not chewing food thoroughly can all exacerbate bloating and gas. Make a concerted effort to eat calmly and mindfully, focusing on eating and savoring each bite. This detailed tracking and thoughtful experimentation can help you make informed decisions that enhance your gut health, improve comfort and overall well-being, and make you feel more engaged and connected to your body's needs.

SKIN ISSUES LINKED TO GUT HEALTH

Have you ever wondered why your skin flares when you need it to look its best? The answer might be lurking in your gut. The gut-skin axis is a fascinating concept. It reveals how closely our gut health is connected to our skin's condition. Imagine your gut and skin as teammates working together toward a common goal: well-being. When your gut is out of balance, it can send distress signals that manifest as skin inflammation. This connection is primarily due to the gut microbiota, the trillions of beneficial and harmful microorganisms in your digestive tract. These tiny organisms influence skin health by modulating inflammation and interacting with the immune system. So, when something goes wrong in your gut, your skin might be the first to show it.

Again, diet plays a significant role in this gut-skin relationship. What you eat can either support or sabotage your skin health. A diet full of sugars and processed foods can disrupt your gut microbiome, leading to imbalances that might trigger skin issues. On the other hand, a diet rich in whole foods and nutrients can nourish your gut and, in turn, improve your skin. Just like feeding your gut the right foods helps it thrive, the same principle applies to your skin. By choosing anti-inflammatory foods, you support your gut and fight your skin against flare-ups.

Several common skin conditions are often linked to gut imbalances. Acne, for instance, is one of the most prevalent skin issues that can be influenced by gut health. When your gut microbiota is disrupted, it can lead to higher inflammation, which may contribute to acne development. Similarly, eczema is characterized by itchy and inflamed skin and has been associated with gut health. I mentioned the concept of a "leaky gut" when the intestinal lining is more permeable; letting unwanted substances enter the bloodstream can exacerbate eczema symptoms. Rosacea, another inflammatory skin condition, can also be affected by gut dysbiosis. These skin issues highlight the importance of maintaining a balanced gut for unblemished, healthier skin.

Improving skin health through the gut involves making mindful dietary and lifestyle changes. Incorporating anti-inflammatory foods with lots of omega-3 fatty acids can be highly beneficial. Foods like salmon, walnuts, and flaxseeds are excellent sources of omega-3s. They can help reduce inflammation, supporting gut and skin health. Staying hydrated is another crucial factor. Water helps maintain skin elasticity. It also flushes out toxins from the body, aiding overall skin and gut health. Think of hydration as a simple yet effective tool in your skincare arsenal, keeping your skin fresh and your gut functioning optimally.

Case studies can often provide the most compelling evidence of the gut-skin relationship. Take Lisa, for example, who struggled with persistent acne for years. After learning about the connection between her gut and skin, she focused on her gut health. Lisa began incorporating more probiotic-rich foods, such as yogurt and fermented vegetables, into her diet. Over several months, she noticed a significant reduction in her acne flare-ups. Her skin became smoother and more vibrant, all thanks to the positive changes she made to support her gut. Lisa's experience is a testament to the power of addressing gut health for improved skin outcomes. It shows that nurturing your gut can pave the way for healthier, more radiant skin.

FATIGUE AND GUT MICROBIOTA: FINDING THE LINK

Imagine you wake up after a whole night's sleep, expecting to feel refreshed and ready to tackle the day, but instead, you struggle to shake off a persistent fog and a sense of exhaustion. This unexplained fatigue might be more than just a poor night's rest—it could be linked to your gut health. The connection between your gut and energy levels is profound and often overlooked. The bacteria in your gut have a crucial role in nutrient absorption, which is vital for fueling your body. When your gut is out of balance, it can struggle to absorb the vitamins and minerals needed to keep your energy levels up, leading to persistent fatigue. Additionally, your gut health influences mitochondrial function, the powerhouses of your cells that produce energy. An imbalance in your gut can hinder these cellular engines, leaving you drained and struggling to concentrate.

Signs that your fatigue may be gut-related can sometimes be subtle. You might feel tired despite getting ample sleep or experience frequent brain fog, making it hard to focus or remember things. These symptoms can often be dismissed as part of a busy lifestyle, but they may indicate that your gut needs attention. When your gut is not functioning at its best, it can lead to systemic issues that manifest as low energy and mental sluggishness. Understanding these signs helps determine the underlying cause of your fatigue and take action to resolve it.

Boosting your energy through gut health involves making targeted dietary and lifestyle changes. Start changing your diet by including complex carbohydrates such as whole grains, legumes, and vegetables. These foods give a steady release of energy, preventing the peaks and crashes associated with simple sugars. Again, regular physical activity is another crucial component. Exercise enhances gut motility, helping food move smoothly through your digestive tract, and increases energy levels by boosting circulation and endorphins. Even a daily brisk walk makes a noticeable difference in how energized you feel.

Certain nutrients are vital for energy production, and gut health can affect absorption. B vitamins, for example, are essential for converting food into energy. If your gut is imbalanced, it may struggle to absorb these vitamins effectively, leaving you feeling fatigued. Ensuring enough B vitamins in your diet or supplements can support your energy levels.

Animal proteins like salmon, eggs, and beef provide B6, B12, and B2, which aid digestion and help beneficial gut bacteria break down nutrients. Plant-based sources like legumes, leafy greens, and brown rice contain B1, B9, and B3, which support energy conversion, feed healthy gut bacteria, and maintain intestinal lining integrity. Fermented foods like nutritional yeast are particularly beneficial, as they combine B vitamins with probiotics to enhance nutrient absorption and gut flora diversity.

Iron is another vital nutrient that transports oxygen throughout your body. A healthy gut aids in iron absorption, ensuring your cells have the oxygen they need to function optimally. Including iron-rich foods like spinach, lentils, and lean meats in your meals can help sustain your energy. Animal sources containing heme iron (red meat, organ meats, and shellfish) are readily absorbed in the gut. However, they should be balanced with fiber-rich foods to prevent digestive discomfort and support beneficial bacteria. Plant-based iron sources like legumes, leafy greens, and seeds provide iron and prebiotic fiber that nourishes gut flora.

The gut's ability to absorb iron depends heavily on overall digestive health and the presence of complementary nutrients. Combining iron-rich foods with vitamin C enhances absorption while maintaining a healthy gut environment. However, certain compounds like tannins in tea and coffee can bind to iron and reduce absorption, so timing these beverages between meals supports optimal gut function and iron uptake.

Consider how you can implement these changes into your daily routine. Let us start with a breakfast rich in complex carbs and B vitamins, like oatmeal topped with nuts and berries. Incorporate a short exercise session in your day, perhaps a walk during your lunch break. Pair iron-rich proteins with vitamin C and fermented foods in simple combinations for a gut-friendly energy boost. Try grilled chicken with sautéed spinach and sweet potatoes, brightened with kimchi and a lemon squeeze. Or keep it light with baked salmon over quinoa, paired with broccoli and sauerkraut, finished with pumpkin seeds and fresh orange segments. Remember to save your coffee or tea between meals to maximize iron absorption.

These adjustments, though simple, can significantly impact your energy levels and overall well-being. Keep in mind that improving your gut health is a gradual process. Be patient with yourself as you make these changes, and pay attention to how your energy and concentration improve over time. Your gut is a powerful ally in maintaining vitality, and by nurturing it, you can experience a renewed sense of energy and focus.

DIGESTIVE DISCOMFORT: DECODING YOUR SYMPTOMS

We have all had those days when our digestive system seemed more like a rollercoaster than a well-tuned engine. You might find yourself dealing with constipation, diarrhea, or the fiery sensation of acid reflux, each bringing its unique challenges. These common digestive discomforts are more than just annoyances—they can reflect your gut's current state of health. Constipation often arises from low fiber intake, where the lack of dietary roughage slows down your intestines. Without enough fiber, your digestive system does not get the bulk it needs to keep things moving smoothly. Conversely, diarrhea can be triggered by infections, certain medications, or an imbalance in gut bacteria. Then, there is acid reflux, usually brought on by certain foods that relax the lower esophageal sphincter, allowing stomach acid to sneak up the esophagus. Foods like spicy dishes, chocolate, or caffeine can be the usual suspects. These issues can disrupt your day and signal underlying gut health concerns.

Recognizing the patterns in your digestive discomfort is key to managing it effectively. Once again, keeping a food and symptom diary can be a game changer. By jotting down what you eat and any symptoms that follow, you can start to identify connections between your diet and your discomfort. You may notice that a particular meal consistently leads to discomfort or that stress makes your symptoms flare up. Stress is a notorious gut disruptor, often leading to digestive issues. Identifying these stress-related triggers can help you take proactive steps to manage your symptoms. With a clearer picture of what is happening, you can make informed diet and lifestyle choices to support your gut health.

Managing digestive discomfort often involves a few strategic adjustments. For acid reflux, small dietary changes can make a big difference. Consider reducing your intake of trigger foods like garlic, onions, and citrus fruits. Eat more frequent, smaller meals rather than large ones to prevent reflux. For constipation, increasing your fiber intake is crucial. Foods like vegetables, fruits, and whole grains add bulk to your diet, promoting regular bowel movements. Drink lots of water because hydration is vital in aiding fiber's smooth transit through your digestive system. While seemingly simple, these adjustments can offer significant relief and support a healthier gut.

While many digestive problems can be dealt with lifestyle changes, knowing when to seek professional help is essential. Never ignore severe or persistent symptoms. If you find that your discomfort continues despite your best efforts, or if you experience symptoms like severe pain, unexplained weight loss, or blood in your stool, it is time to consult a healthcare professional. These could be signs of more serious conditions that require medical evaluation. The impact on your quality of life is also a crucial factor. If your symptoms interrupt your daily activities or cause significant distress, seeking professional guidance can provide clarity and relief. It is always better to address these issues sooner rather than later, ensuring you receive the appropriate care and support for your gut health.

UNDERSTANDING FOOD ALLERGIES AND INTOLERANCES

Your body might signal food sensitivities if your stomach churns after eating certain foods or you experience unexpected symptoms like headaches or skin rashes. These reactions can cause anything from minor discomfort to terrible allergic responses, and understanding the difference is crucial for maintaining optimal gut health. Your digestive system's response to different foods can give vital insights into your overall health, and learning to interpret these signals can transform your well-being.

Common Food Triggers

The most frequent food triggers that affect gut health include gluten, dairy products, eggs, soy, tree nuts, peanuts, shellfish, and certain fruits. These foods can cause reactions in sensitive individuals due to their protein structures or natural compounds.

For instance, gluten in wheat, barley, and rye can trigger reactions ranging from mild sensitivity to severe celiac disease. Dairy products containing lactose often cause digestive issues in those lacking sufficient lactase enzyme. Understanding these common triggers helps you identify potential problem foods in your diet and take appropriate action to protect your gut health.

Difference Between Allergy and Intolerance

Food allergies and intolerances might seem similar, but they involve different mechanisms within your body. A food allergy initiates an immune system response, often immediate and potentially severe, involving immunoglobulin E (IgE) antibodies. Your body treats the food as a threat, leading to symptoms like hives, difficulty breathing, or, in severe cases, anaphylaxis. On the other hand, food intolerances typically involve the digestive system and occur when your body cannot properly break down certain foods. These reactions are usually less severe but can cause significant discomfort through symptoms like bloating, gas, diarrhea, or constipation. The timeline of symptoms often helps distinguish between the two—allergic reactions typically occur within minutes to hours, while intolerances may take longer to manifest.

Testing and Diagnosis

Identifying food allergies and intolerances requires a systematic approach, often involving medical testing and careful observation. Your healthcare provider might recommend skin prick or blood tests measuring specific IgE antibodies for suspected food allergies. These tests can help pinpoint exactly which foods trigger your immune system. Food intolerances can be more challenging to diagnose, often requiring an elimination diet where you temporarily remove suspected trigger foods and gradually reintroduce them while monitoring your symptoms. This process, though time-consuming, provides valuable information about your body's responses to specific foods.

Modern diagnostic tools have expanded our understanding of food sensitivities. Specialized tests can now measure enzyme levels, such as lactase for dairy intolerance, or assess celiac disease markers through blood work and intestinal biopsies. However, it is essential to remember that not all food sensitivity tests are equally reliable, and some popular commercial tests lack scientific validation. Working with healthcare professionals who understand both traditional and emerging diagnostic methods ensures you receive accurate information about your food sensitivities.

Identifying and managing food allergies and intolerances often requires patience and dedication. Many people find that keeping a detailed food diary helps track symptoms and identify patterns. This information becomes invaluable when working with healthcare providers to develop an appropriate management plan. Additionally, understanding your specific triggers allows you to make informed decisions about your diet while ensuring you maintain proper nutrition through suitable alternatives. Remember that food sensitivities can change over time, so regular reassessment of your tolerances may be necessary.

WEIGHT FLUCTUATIONS: IS YOUR GUT TO BLAME?

Think about the last time you stepped on the scale and noticed a change in your weight that seemed to come out of nowhere. This can be frustrating if you have not changed your eating and exercise habits. Your gut health might be more prominent in this fluctuation than you realize. The microorganisms in your gut, known as the gut microbiota, are key players in how your body processes and stores fat. These tiny organisms influence your metabolism by decomposing complex carbohydrates and generating SCFA, which your body uses for energy. This process can affect how much fat your body stores. This process can affect how much fat your body stores. If your gut bacteria are out of balance, it might increase fat storage and weight gain.

A diverse gut microbiome, which includes a wide variety of beneficial bacteria, is generally associated with a healthy weight. However, when this microbial diversity decreases, as it often does with a diet high in processed foods and low in fiber, it can contribute to obesity. This lack of diversity might reduce your body's ability to effectively regulate fat storage and energy extraction from food. Studies have suggested that those with obesity often have a gut microbiome less diverse than those with a healthy weight. This link highlights the importance of maintaining a balanced and varied microbiome for weight management.

If you are experiencing rapid weight changes without altering your lifestyle or finding it difficult to lose weight despite a healthy diet, your gut health may be part of the problem. These signs suggest that your gut might not function optimally due to an imbalance in your gut bacteria. This imbalance can disrupt your metabolism and lead to weight fluctuations. It is essential to consider the health of your gut when addressing these issues, as it plays a crucial role in how your body manages weight.

Add fiber-rich foods to your meals to achieve a healthy weight through improved gut health. Foods like whole grains, beans, and fruits provide the necessary bulk to promote satiety, helping you feel full and satisfied longer. This can naturally reduce your calorie intake without the need for strict dieting. At the same time, it is crucial to avoid processed foods that can disrupt your gut balance. These foods often have preservatives and additives that negatively affect your gut microbiome, reducing its diversity and efficiency. Focusing on whole, unprocessed foods supports a healthier gut environment and a more stable weight.

Research and success stories further illustrate the connection between gut health and weight management. For instance, studies show that probiotics can be prominent in weight loss and maintenance. Certain probiotic strains have been found to influence body weight and fat mass, helping people achieve their weight goals. These beneficial bacteria can improve gut health by increasing microbial diversity and enhancing metabolic functions. Probiotics may not be a magic solution, but they can be valuable in your weight management arsenal. By incorporating them into your diet, you may find it easier to manage your weight and maintain a healthy balance.

Understanding the link between your gut and weight offers a new perspective on weight management. Rather than focusing solely on calories or exercise, consider the impact that your gut health may have. By nurturing your microbiome through dietary choices and lifestyle habits, you support your body's natural ability to manage weight effectively. These insights into gut health and weight regulation offer a fresh take on achieving and maintaining a healthy weight, reminding us that our bodies are intricately connected systems that thrive on balance. As we move forward, we will explore how these connections extend to other areas of health and well-being. We will underscore the importance of a holistic approach to nurturing our guts.

CHAPTER 4

BUILDING GUT-FRIENDLY HABITS

A t times, meals were a mere race for me, a moment to get through rather than savor. I often wolfed down lunch between meetings or gulped a quick breakfast in the car, leaving me feeling bloated and sluggish. It was not until I stumbled upon the concept of mindful eating that everything changed. The simple act of being present and attentive during meals revolutionized my digestion and my relationship with food. Conscious eating, in stark contrast to my previous habits, is about slowing down, savoring each bite, and truly being in the moment with your meal. It is a practice that invites you to appreciate food for more than just its nutritional value, connecting you to the experience of eating in a satisfying and nourishing way. This chapter will explore simple, everyday habits you can change to improve your gut health.

INTRODUCTION TO MINDFUL EATING

Mindful eating begins with creating an environment that encourages you to focus on your meal. Start with a quiet, calming space free from distractions like phones or televisions, where you can fully engage with your food. Then, as you eat, begin by noticing your meal's colors, textures, and aromas. As you take each bite, pay attention to the flavors and how they change as you chew. This process enhances enjoyment and helps your body recognize when your stomach is full, preventing overeating. Recognizing hunger and fullness cues is an essential aspect of mindful eating. It encourages you to listen to your body—eat when you are truly hungry, and stop when satisfied—an approach that naturally supports a healthy gut.

The benefits of conscious eating extend far beyond the meal itself. By reducing your eating pace, you can significantly decrease the stress on your digestive system. This practice promotes better digestion, as taking your time allows digestive enzymes to do their job more efficiently. As a result, you may experience less bloating and discomfort after meals. But that is not all. Mindful eating also enhances nutrient absorption, enabling your body to make the most of your foods. Studies show that mindful eating can reduce IBS symptoms and improve gut health. For example, the one published in the Journal of Gastroenterology found that participants who practiced mindful eating experienced a significant reduction in IBS symptoms. It is a simple yet powerful way to boost your gut health while cultivating a deeper appreciation for the food on your plate.

By practicing mindful eating daily, you are changing eating

habits and taking control of your health. Start by setting aside a few minutes before each meal to take a deep breath and center yourself. This small ritual can help shift your focus from the day's stresses to the meal before you. Engage your senses by savoring the texture of your food, the crunch of a fresh apple, or the silkiness of yogurt. These sensory experiences make eating more enjoyable and satisfying, turning a routine meal into a moment of mindfulness. Over time, these practices become second nature, helping you develop a more intuitive relationship with food and your body's needs. This empowerment is a key aspect of mindful eating, allowing you to make deliberate, healthy choices about your diet.

Reflection Section: Embracing Mindful Eating

Consider embarking on a transformative exercise during your next meal: deliberately put your fork aside between each bite and chew your food slowly, savoring the complexity of flavors and textures. Engage deeply with how your body responds to each morsel. Do you notice moments of satisfaction or a sense of fullness that might ordinarily be overlooked in the haste of daily life? This exercise invites you to reflect on these sensations and their impact on your eating habits. Maintaining a journal of these mindful eating experiences can illuminate your relationship with food, uncovering patterns that either bolster or detract from your gut health. This practice does not just aid digestion—it empowers you to make deliberate, healthy choices about your diet.

To illustrate the profound impact of mindful eating, consider the story of James, a dedicated professional whose fast-paced lifestyle led to persistent digestive discomfort. The constant rush meant meals were often consumed hastily, without pausing to genuinely appreciate the food before him. The decision to embrace mindful eating—slowing down, fully experiencing each bite, and acknowledging the flavors and textures—significantly shifted James's digestive health and overall mood. This subtle yet powerful change in approach allowed James to attune to his body's hunger and fullness signals more accurately, fostering a more balanced and harmonious eating routine. James's experience is a compelling testament to the transformative power of mindful eating—the idea that dedicating time to be present with our meals can instigate meaningful improvements in our health and well-being, even amid the relentless pace of modern life. Stories like James's inspire us all to make similar changes in our lives, embracing the transformative power of mindful eating.

STRESS-REDUCTION TECHNIQUES FOR GUT HEALTH

As I have pointed out in previous chapters, stress is one of those sneaky factors that can quietly wreak havoc on your gut. When life's demands pile up and stress becomes a constant companion, it can disrupt the delicate balance of your gut health. Chronic stress is not just a mental game—it affects your body profoundly, mainly your gut. Your digestive system operates under the influence of the enteric nervous system, often called the "second brain," which is closely linked to stress levels. When stress is chronic, it activates the hypothalamic-pituitary-adrenal (HPA) axis, leading to increased inflammation and impaired digestive function. Your gut motility, the rate food moves through your digestive tract, can become erratic. This may lead to problems like IBS or dysbiosis, where the balance of harmful and good bacteria in your gut is thrown off. You may remember that stress also influences gut permeability, potentially leading to a "leaky gut," where dangerous substances can pass through the gut lining, causing inflammation.

Fortunately, there are simple, effective ways to combat stress and protect your gut health, like adding stress-reduction techniques to your daily routine, which can be transformative. Breathing exercises are a straightforward yet powerful way to calm your nervous system. Taking slow, deep breaths activates the parasympathetic nervous system, which helps counteract stress. Progressive muscle relaxation is another easy-to-use technique. It is tensing, then relaxing muscle groups in your body, promoting a sense of calm and easing tension. These can be easily incorporated into your day at work or home. Short mindfulness breaks during work hours can also make a significant difference. Taking a few minutes to step away from your desk and focus on your breath or a calming image can reset your stress levels. Establishing a wind-down routine in the evening can also help prepare you for restful sleep. This might include gentle stretches, a warm bath, or listening to soothing music. The simplicity of these techniques makes managing stress and protecting your gut health achievable for everyone.

Integrating these techniques into a busy schedule might seem challenging, but it is all about finding moments of calm amid the chaos. Start by setting aside five minutes daily for a breathing exercise or mindfulness practice. You could do this in the morning to set a positive tone for the day or during a lunch break to recharge. You can gradually extend the time you dedicate to these practices as you become more comfortable with them. Evening routines are equally important. Consider creating a relaxation ritual, such as reading a book or journaling before bed, to signal your body that it is time to unwind. Over weeks and months, these small changes can add up, reducing stress and supporting gut health.

The research underscores the benefits of stress reduction for gut health. Studies show that mindfulness practices can improve gut function by promoting parasympathetic nervous system dominance, which is beneficial for digestion. For instance, one study reviewed in "Mindful Eating: A Review of How the Stress-Digestion-Mindfulness Triad May Modulate and Improve Gastrointestinal and Digestive Function" highlights how mindfulness can help regulate stress responses, improving overall wellness. Real-life examples further illustrate these benefits. Take Frankie, a busy professional who struggled with stress-induced IBS. She saw a significant reduction in her symptoms by adding breathing exercises and progressive muscle relaxation into her routine. Emily found that even short moments of mindfulness throughout her day helped her manage stress and support her gut health. Her experience shows that with dedication, stress-reduction techniques can seamlessly integrate into even the busiest lives. These practices alleviate stress and enhance your body's resilience, allowing your gut to function optimally.

MEAL PLANNING FOR THE BUSY INDIVIDUAL

In a world where time is often our most limited resource, meal planning emerges as a real hope for those striving to maintain a balanced diet amid the chaos. I used to find myself grabbing whatever was quick and easy, usually processed and far from gut-friendly. But then I realized that with some planning, I could ensure a steady intake of the nutrients my gut needed to thrive. Planning meals helps you avoid relying on convenience foods that are often high in preservatives and low in nutrition. Instead, it allows you to focus on incorporating a variety of gut-friendly nutrients, such as fiber, probiotics, and healthy fats, which are crucial for maintaining a healthy microbiota.

For those who are perpetually on the go, meal planning does not have to be daunting. Begin with batch cooking, a strategy where you prepare large quantities of food in advance and store them in the freezer for future use. This approach saves time and ensures you have nutritious meals ready. Consider creating a weekly meal template to simplify the process. This template can serve as a blueprint, guiding your grocery shopping and meal preparation. Having a plan reduces decision fatigue and makes sticking to your gut health goals more manageable.

When it comes to meal ideas, simplicity is key, especially on busy days. Overnight oats are a perfect example—mix oats with your choice of yogurt, milk, or kefir, add some berries and seeds, and let them sit in the fridge overnight. In the morning, you have a nutritious breakfast ready to go. Quinoa salad with mixed vegetables and chickpeas is another quick and easy option. Prepare a large batch and enjoy it the whole week. It is packed with fiber and protein, satisfying and nourishing your gut. These meals are not only easy to prepare but also offer the variety that your microbiome thrives on.

Consider leveraging technology to streamline your meal-planning efforts. Numerous apps and tools are designed to make meal planning a breeze. Apps like Mealime or Tasty can help you organize your meals, generate grocery lists, and even provide cooking inspiration. These tools are handy for those with hectic schedules, offering a convenient way to stay on top of your meal planning. With these resources, you can transform meal planning from a chore into an enjoyable and rewarding habit.

Interactive Element: Weekly Meal Template

Creating a visual weekly meal template can help keep your meal planning organized and stress-free. Outline a simple chart on a piece of paper, or use a digital planner to outline your meals for each day of the week. Include breakfast, lunch, dinner, and snacks. Fill in your template with ideas based on the ingredients you have or plan to purchase. Consider incorporating themes like "Meatless Mondays" or "Soup Sundays" to add variety and make planning easier. This template is a visual reminder of your goals and helps you stay committed to supporting your gut health through thoughtful meal choices.

Meal planning for gut health is about organization and setting yourself up for success. By planning, you create a structure that makes it easier to make healthy choices, even on your busiest days.

This proactive approach empowers you to take control of your diet and provides the foundation for a thriving gut. With dedication and the right tools, meal planning can become a manageable and rewarding part of your routine.

COOKING AT HOME: SIMPLE GUT-FRIENDLY RECIPES

There is something wonderfully liberating about cooking at home. It grants you the power to choose fresh, whole ingredients and control portion sizes vital for gut health. Unlike dining out, where you often face a mystery of hidden sugars, unhealthy fats, and oversized portions, cooking in your kitchen lets you tailor every dish to your needs. This control allows you to experiment with new gut-friendly recipes, exploring flavors and textures that delight the palate and nourish the microbiome. Imagine the joy of knowing exactly what goes into your meals—each ingredient chosen with care and intent.

Basic cooking techniques are your best allies in this endeavor, helping you preserve nutrients while enhancing digestion. Steaming vegetables is an excellent way to keep their vitamins intact while making them easier for your gut to process, like a plate of vibrant broccoli, tender yet crisp, retaining all its natural goodness. Roasting can also transform root vegetables like sweet potatoes and carrots into caramelized delights that are both nourishing and satisfying. This adds a depth of flavor that steaming might not, giving you variety in textures and tastes. Then, the art of preparing fermented foods, such as kimchi or yogurt. These are rich in probiotics, those beneficial bacteria that support a healthy gut flora. Fermentation is a time-honored tradition that turns simple ingredients into powerful allies for your digestive system, offering your gut the diverse population of microbes it thrives on.

To make the most of cooking at home, let us dive into a couple of simple, delicious recipes. Start with a hearty lentil soup featuring spinach and turmeric. Lentils are an excellent source of fiber and protein, while turmeric offers anti-inflammatory benefits, making this soup a gut-friendly powerhouse. Cook lentils with diced carrots and onions, add a dash of turmeric, and finish with fresh spinach for a nutritious meal. Another option is grilled salmon paired with quinoa and roasted vegetables. Salmon provides omega-3 fatty acids, essential for reducing inflammation, while quinoa is a complete protein that complements any dish. Roast a good mix of seasonal vegetables like bell peppers and zucchini alongside the salmon for a colorful, flavorful plate. These meals are simple to prepare and full of nutrients your gut will thank you for.

Cooking at home also invites creativity and personalization. You can change recipes to suit your preferences or dietary needs, allowing you to cater to any intolerances or allergies. If lactose intolerant, swap yogurt with coconut-based alternatives or use almond milk in your recipes. Consider adding spices and herbs not just for flavor but for their health benefits. Cumin and coriander, for instance, can aid digestion, while fresh herbs such as parsley and basil add freshness and vitality to any dish. This flexibility encourages you to play with flavors and create meals that are uniquely yours, ensuring that cooking remains enjoyable and rewarding.

The beauty of cooking at home is the freedom it gives you to nourish your body and soul. It is an opportunity to connect with the food you eat, explore new flavors, and take charge of your health in an empowering and satisfying way. As you experiment with these recipes and techniques, remember that the kitchen is your playground, a space for creativity and growth. Embrace the process, enjoy the results, and relish the benefits of every gut-friendly meal you create.

DINING OUT: MAKING GUT-CONSCIOUS CHOICES

Navigating restaurant menus can feel like a treasure hunt for those looking to maintain gut health. However, with some strategy, you can enjoy dining out without compromising your wellness goals. When scanning a menu, it is wise to opt for grilled or steamed dishes instead of fried options. These cooking methods typically use less oil and retain more of the food's natural nutrients. Grilled fish or chicken paired with vegetables tastes tremendous and supports your gut health by providing lean proteins and fibers. Another tip is to ask for dressings and sauces on the side. This allows you to control how much you consume, reducing unnecessary sugars and fats that can upset your digestive balance. Remember, you have the power to tailor your meal to fit your needs, and most restaurants are happy to accommodate these simple requests.

Communicating your dietary preferences to restaurant staff is crucial, especially if you have specific gut health requirements or food intolerances. Approach your server with politeness and clarity when inquiring about ingredient modifications. For example, you might ask if a dish can be prepared without dairy or with extra vegetables instead of bread. Informing staff of any allergies or intolerances upfront ensures that your meal is prepared safely and to your liking. It is often helpful to explain briefly the reason for your request, as this can foster understanding and cooperation. Many people in the food industry are used to accommodating various dietary needs and will do their best to ensure your dining experience is enjoyable and safe.

Dining out presents challenges, but you can avoid pitfalls with some foresight. One effective strategy is managing portion sizes by sharing dishes with a dining partner or taking half of your meal home as leftovers. This approach helps prevent overeating and allows you to enjoy a wider variety of flavors without feeling overindulgent. Choosing water or herbal tea over sugary beverages is another simple way to stay on track. These drinks are refreshing and hydrating without the added sugars that cause spikes in blood sugar and affect your energy levels. Considering these strategies, you can enjoy your meal while supporting your gut health.

Let us look at a few stories of those who have successfully maintained their gut health while dining out. Take Sophie, for instance. She loves dining out with friends but used to feel anxious about making gut-friendly restaurant choices. She started by researching menus online before arriving, which gave her time to plan her meal and feel confident in her selections. Eventually, Sophie found a balance that allowed her to enjoy her favorite restaurants without compromising her gut health. Her experience shows that dining out can be a delightful and stress-free experience with some preparation and communication.

Similarly, Tom discovered that by sticking to his principles of choosing grilled over fried and requesting sauces on the side, he could indulge in dining out without the usual digestive discomfort that followed. His willingness to speak up about his preferences and make mindful choices has allowed him to enjoy meals with friends and family while maintaining his health goals. Stories like these demonstrate that dining out can seamlessly integrate into a gut-healthy lifestyle with thoughtful consideration and a proactive approach.

CHAPTER 5

DIETARY CHANGES FOR A HEALTHY GUT

One chilly morning, I stared at a bowl of vibrant, fresh vegetables—kale, radishes, and beets glistening with dew. I was at a local farmer's market, drawn in by the sight of these whole foods in their purest form. It struck me how powerful these simple foods could transform our health. Whole foods, those unprocessed and nutrient-rich gems like vegetables, whole grains, fresh fruits, seeds, and nuts, can be the foundation of a healthy gut. They are rich in vital vitamins, minerals, and antioxidants that our bodies crave, acting as natural fuel for our daily lives. When we fill our plates with whole foods, we nourish ourselves and support the community of beneficial bacteria in our gut that is vital for maintaining balance and health.

STEPS TOWARD A BALANCED WHOLE-FOOD DIET

Whole foods are the unsung heroes of a balanced diet that has a good variety of foods in the proper proportions. A balanced diet is crucial because it ensures you get all your body's nutrients. Whole foods are a key part of this. Unlike processed foods that often strip away vital components, whole foods retain their natural goodness. They are loaded with fiber, a key element for digestion, acting like a gentle broom that sweeps through your digestive tract, keeping things moving smoothly. This fiber also serves as a prebiotic. It feeds your gut's beneficial bacteria and promotes a healthy microbiome. The nutrient density of whole foods supports overall health, providing a steady stream of energy without the crashes and spikes associated with sugary snacks. This stability is not only good for your waistline but also for your mental clarity and focus.

Imagine a rainbow of fresh fruits and vegetables when you think of whole foods. These vibrant colors are not just eye-catching; they are indicators of the antioxidants and phytonutrients packed within. Whole grains like quinoa and brown rice are another excellent choice, offering complex carbohydrates that provide sustained energy. Seeds and nuts like chia and almonds are small but mighty, delivering healthy fats and protein. These foods are delicious and essential for a thriving gut microbiome. Incorporating them into your diet lays a solid foundation for your health, supporting everything from digestion to immune function.

Transitioning to a whole-food diet is more straightforward than it may seem. Start by making small, manageable changes. For example, you can swap refined grains for whole grains in your meals. This simple switch can dramatically increase fiber intake, supporting digestion and satiety. You can also add various colorful produce to your plate. Each color represents different nutrients, so eating a spectrum ensures you get a wide range of vitamins and minerals. Remember, it is about progress, not perfection.

Navigating dietary changes can often feel like navigating a complex maze, filled with obstacles such as unfamiliarity with whole foods or a packed schedule that leaves little room for meal prep. As mentioned in the previous chapter, planning meals can be a game changer. Spend a little time mapping out your meals each week to avoid the temptation of processed options. This strategic investment of time can streamline your week and ensure you always have access to nutritious meals.

Begin by choosing recipes that match your health goals, then create a shopping list to keep your grocery trips efficient and focused. Cooking in bulk is another savvy approach to managing your time and ensuring healthy meals are ready, even on your busiest days. Dishes that freeze well, such as casseroles, stews, and soups, can be prepared in large quantities and stored for later use. This method reduces daily cooking time and the temptation to reach for less healthy, processed options when pressed for time.

Understanding food labels is a powerful skill. Look for products that list whole foods as their main ingredients, and avoid those with a long list of additives. When buying ingredients, spend a few extra minutes reading labels carefully. This practice can dramatically enhance your understanding of whole-food options and help you avoid products laden with unnecessary additives and preservatives. Knowledge is power, and being able to discern the quality of the ingredients you use empowers you to make choices that are in harmony with your wellness objectives.

Integrating these strategies into your lifestyle can smooth the transition to a whole-food diet, minimizing the feeling of overhaul and making the process feel like a natural evolution. This gentle approach is less about perfection from the outset and more about making consistent, informed choices that nourish and balance your gut health and overall well-being.

Interactive Element: Whole-Food Challenge

Consider embarking on a weekly "Whole-Food Exploration Challenge." Select one whole food you have never tried or seldom included in your diet each week. Document this journey in a designated journal, detailing the food chosen, how you decided to prepare it, and any observations you make about its impact on your well-being. This could include changes in digestion, energy levels, or even mood. Consciously integrating new, unprocessed foods into your meals encourages a culinary adventure, inviting you to savor unfamiliar flavors and textures. Remember, it is not about restriction but expanding your culinary horizons.

As time passes, this challenge diversifies your palate and strengthens your gut health, potentially leading to noticeable improvements in overall wellness. Moreover, this practice fosters a meaningful engagement with your dietary habits, making the shift toward whole foods a rewarding and enlightening experience that deepens your connection to the food on your plate. Through this approach, you will likely uncover new favorite dishes that enhance your health while expanding your culinary repertoire, making each meal an opportunity for discovery and delight.

FERMENTED FOODS: ADDING PROBIOTICS NATURALLY

Once upon a time, my curiosity about gut health led me to a small, bustling market stall brimming with jars of vibrant, fermented foods. I began appreciating how these foods could transform a meal and our gut health. Through the magic of natural processes, fermented foods become rich in probiotics. These beneficial bacteria, like lactobacillus found in yogurt, help maintain our gut microbiomes' healthy balances. Fermentation is a time-tested method that enhances food by promoting the growth of good bacteria. During fermentation, bacteria and yeast convert sugars in food into acids or alcohol, creating an environment where beneficial microbes thrive. This preserves the food and enhances its nutritional value, supporting a diverse and balanced microbiome.

You will find a delightful array while exploring the world of fermented foods. Sauerkraut and kimchi, both made from fermented cabbage, offer a tangy crunch that is perfect for adding to meals. Miso, a traditional Japanese paste made from fermented soybeans, is another versatile ingredient that can bring depth to soups and marinades. Kombucha, a fizzy fermented tea, is both refreshing and probiotic-rich, making it a popular beverage choice. Kefir, similar to yogurt, is a cultured dairy product with a thinner consistency. It is a fantastic addition to smoothies or enjoyed independently. These foods introduce beneficial bacteria into your system and add unique textures and flavors to your diet, making healthy eating an enjoyable adventure.

Incorporating fermented foods into your meals does not have to be complicated. Add a spoonful of kimchi to rice bowls or salads for an easy flavor boost. Its spicy, tangy profile complements various dishes, adding taste and probiotic benefits. Yogurt is another versatile option. Blend fruits and honey into a smoothie base for a nutritious, gut-friendly snack. These small additions can enhance your meals and give your gut the probiotics it needs to flourish.

For those who enjoy experimenting in the kitchen, making fermented foods at home can be a rewarding experience. Start with something simple, like sauerkraut. All you need is cabbage and salt. Shred the cabbage finely, sprinkle it with salt, and massage it until it releases its juices. Pack it tightly into a jar, submerging the cabbage in its liquid, and let it ferment at room temperature for a week or two. The result is a tangy, crunchy condiment that can elevate your meals and support your gut health.

Fermenting pickles is another easy project for home enthusiasts. Using fresh cucumbers and dill, you can create a batch of pickles that are not only delicious but also filled with probiotics. Slice the cucumbers, place them in a jar with dill and garlic, and cover them with a saltwater brine. Allow them to ferment for a few days until they reach your desired level of tanginess. The process is simple and fun, offering a sense of accomplishment as you create probiotic-rich foods. Home fermentation allows you to connect with your food more profoundly, understanding the life cycle from raw ingredients to a nourishing addition to your diet.

Avoiding Common Gut Irritants

In the quest for better gut health, it is crucial to recognize the culprits that might be causing havoc in your digestive system. Processed foods, often brimming with additives and preservatives, are one of the main offenders. These ingredients, designed to extend shelf life and enhance flavor, can disrupt your gut's natural balance. Remember that your gut is a delicate ecosystem. Introducing artificial elements can tip the scales, leading to inflammation and discomfort. Similarly, artificial sweeteners like aspartame, often marketed as a healthier alternative to sugar, can have a negative impact. They may alter gut bacteria and potentially lead to bloating or stomach upset for some people. It is worth being mindful of the ingredients in your pantry and opting for natural alternatives whenever possible.

Identifying which foods irritate your gut can feel like solving a mystery. Again, keeping a food diary is an excellent method to track what you eat and how you feel afterward. Documenting meals and related symptoms can help you notice patterns and pinpoint potential triggers. Perhaps you always feel bloated after eating a particular type of bread or experience discomfort after drinking a specific beverage. Noticing these connections empowers you to make informed decisions about your diet. Everyone's gut is unique, so what troubles one person may not affect another. You can tailor your diet to cater to your needs by tuning into your body's signals.

Once you have identified your irritants, exploring healthier alternatives can be a joyful journey of discovery. If soda is your go-to refreshment, consider switching to herbal teas or infused water. These options can be just as refreshing and satisfying without the added sugars and chemicals. Infuse water with slices of citrus or cucumber to provide flavor and hydration. When it comes to fruit juices, opt for whole fruits instead. Whole fruits offer fiber, which aids digestion and helps you feel full, unlike their juiced counterparts. By making these swaps, you support your gut while enjoying delicious flavors.

Alcohol and caffeine, though popular, can also pose challenges for gut health. Alcohol, especially in excess, can harm the gut lining and disrupt the balance of bacteria. Meanwhile, caffeine, while providing that much-needed energy boost, can sometimes lead to acid reflux or an upset stomach if consumed in large amounts. Moderation is key with these substances. Try limiting your intake and choosing gut-friendly options when possible. For instance, if you are a coffee lover, consider caffeine-free alternatives like chicory root coffee. It offers a similar taste profile without the caffeine, making it a gentler choice for your gut.

It is all about finding what works for you. While these suggestions provide a starting point, the journey to gut health is personal. Experiment with different foods and drinks, paying attention to how your body responds. This will help you cultivate a diet that nourishes your gut and aligns with your tastes and lifestyle.

EVIDENCE-BASED DIETARY PROTOCOLS

Navigating the world of therapeutic diets can feel overwhelming, especially when you are seeking relief from digestive issues. While many dietary approaches claim to improve gut health, some have more substantial scientific backing than others. Understanding these evidence-based protocols can help you decide which approach might work best for your situation. Remember that while these diets can be powerful tools for healing, they are most effective when implemented under proper guidance and with a clear understanding of their principles.

Understanding the Low-FODMAP Diet

The low-FODMAP diet has emerged as one of the most well-researched approaches to managing digestive symptoms, particularly in IBS cases. As discussed, FODMAPs are poorly absorbed carbohydrates in the small intestine, leading to digestive distress in sensitive individuals. These compounds are found in various foods, from garlic and onions to certain fruits and dairy products. When these foods reach the large intestine undigested, they can be fermented by gut bacteria, potentially causing bloating, gas, and other uncomfortable symptoms.

This diet's protocol involves three distinct phases: elimination, reintroduction, and personalization. During the elimination phase, which typically lasts two to six weeks, you remove all high-FODMAP foods from your diet. This gives your digestive system time to calm down and establish a baseline of symptoms. The reintroduction phase systematically brings back one FODMAP group at a time, allowing you to identify specific trigger foods and your personal tolerance levels. This methodical approach helps create a more sustainable, personalized diet that relieves symptoms while maximizing food variety.

Elimination Diet Basics

An elimination diet is a diagnostic tool and potential healing protocol for identifying food sensitivities and reducing inflammation. This approach removes common trigger foods from your diet for a specified period, typically three to four weeks, allowing your body to reset and inflammation to subside. Common foods eliminated include dairy, gluten, soy, eggs, corn, and processed foods. The process requires careful planning to ensure nutritional adequacy while eliminating potential triggers. Many report improved energy levels, better digestion, and reduced symptoms during this phase.

The reintroduction phase of an elimination diet is equally important as the elimination phase. Foods are reintroduced one at a time, usually every three to four days, while carefully monitoring for reactions. This systematic approach helps identify specific foods contributing to your symptoms. It is crucial to keep detailed records during this phase, noting not only obvious digestive symptoms but also changes in energy levels, mood, skin condition, and sleep quality. This information becomes invaluable in creating your long-term dietary plan.

Other Therapeutic Diets

Beyond low-FODMAP and elimination diets, several other evidence-based approaches can support gut health. The specific carbohydrate diet (SCD) has shown promise for inflammatory bowel conditions by eliminating complex carbohydrates and focusing on easily digestible nutrients. This diet works by starving out harmful bacteria. At the same time, it promotes the growth of beneficial gut flora. While not strictly therapeutic, the Mediterranean diet has substantial research supporting its benefits for gut health by emphasizing whole foods, healthy fats, and abundant fiber.

The autoimmune protocol (AIP) represents another systematic approach, particularly beneficial for those with autoimmune conditions affecting the gut. This protocol eliminates potential trigger foods while emphasizing nutrient-dense alternatives that support gut healing. Like an elimination diet, AIP includes a reintroduction phase to identify personal tolerances. The gut-healing diet spectrum also includes modified versions of ketogenic diets, which some research suggests may help reduce gut inflammation and support microbiome diversity.

When considering any therapeutic diet, it is essential to remember that no single meal plan works for everyone. Your individual needs, lifestyle, and health goals should guide your choice of dietary protocol. These diets often require significant commitment and planning, so having proper support and guidance can make the difference between success and frustration. Working with healthcare providers who understand these protocols can help you navigate challenges, ensure nutritional adequacy, and make necessary modifications to suit your situation. As research in nutritional science continues to evolve, new evidence-based approaches may emerge, offering even more options for supporting gut health through dietary intervention.

HYDRATION AND GUT HEALTH: THE OVERLOOKED CONNECTION

I remember overhearing a conversation at the gym about the importance of staying hydrated, and it got me thinking about how often we overlook water's vital role in our digestive health. Water is more than just a thirst-quencher; it is a key player in digestion, supporting nutrient absorption and waste elimination. Imagine water as the lubricant that helps your digestive system run smoothly, ensuring nutrients are absorbed efficiently and waste is flushed out. It also helps preserve the mucosal lining of the intestines, which is a protective barrier. This lining keeps harmful substances at bay while allowing essential nutrients to pass through, a balance crucial for a healthy gut. When you are hydrated, your body can perform these tasks more effectively, reducing the likelihood of constipation or bloating.

Knowing how much water to drink can be confusing. You have probably heard the adage about needing exactly eight glasses daily, but hydration needs vary from person to person. Drinking water consistently throughout the day is generally a good practice. Pay attention to your body's cues; if you feel thirsty, it is a sign you need more fluids. Your water intake should also adjust based on your activity level and climate. If you exercise or are in hot weather, you need more water to replenish what you have lost through sweat. Keeping a reusable water bottle handy can remind you to sip throughout the day, making it easier to stay hydrated without overthinking.

Water is not the only source of hydration. Many foods and beverages can help keep you hydrated, pleasantly contributing to your fluid intake. Water-rich fruits like watermelon and cucumber are fantastic options. They are refreshing and high in water content, making them perfect for a hot day or a light snack. Herbal teas are another excellent choice. Whether you prefer chamomile, mint, or hibiscus, these teas provide hydration without caffeine, which can sometimes have a diuretic effect. Broths, especially homemade ones, are warm and soothing, offering hydration and a dose of nutrients. Including these options in your diet can enhance your hydration routine, adding variety and flavor.

There are plenty of myths about hydration floating around. One common misconception is that drinking water dilutes stomach acids, interfering with digestion. However, water aids digestion by helping break down food. This makes it easier for your body to absorb nutrients. Another myth is that you can only get hydrated by drinking plain water. As we have explored, hydrating foods and other beverages can also contribute significantly to your daily fluid intake. Anticipating the signs of dehydration is crucial for maintaining gut health. If you are feeling lightheaded, have a dry mouth, or notice darker urine, these could signal that you need to increase your water intake. Staying aware of these signs helps you avoid dehydration and supports your digestive system in functioning optimally.

Including more water in your daily routine can be simple and enjoyable. Start your morning with a glass of water, perhaps with a splash of lemon for a zesty kick. This habit not only hydrates you but can also kickstart your metabolism. As you go about your day, drink a glass of water before each meal. This practice can help you feel fuller, potentially aiding in portion control while ensuring you remain well-hydrated. A pitcher of infused water in the fridge, with slices of your favorite fruit or herbs, can make reaching for water more appealing. This small effort can transform hydration from a chore into a refreshing ritual.

BALANCING INDULGENCE WITH GUT HEALTH

Imagine a weekend afternoon in a cozy café with the smell of freshly baked pastries wafting through the air. It is easy to enjoy these moments without guilt, knowing occasional indulgence is part of a balanced, healthy lifestyle. Life is too short to forgo the pleasures of a favorite treat altogether. The key is balance, which allows you to savor these indulgences without compromising your gut health. Remembering that feeling deprived can lead to stress and even overindulgence later is essential. Allowing yourself a treat occasionally helps maintain a positive relationship with food and reduces the guilt often tied to eating certain foods.

Balancing indulgence with gut health involves making mindful choices. One effective strategy is practicing portion control. Instead of diving into a whole cake, enjoy a small slice. This way, you get to indulge without overloading your system. Pairing treats with nutritious meals is another intelligent approach. If you plan to eat dessert, consider preceding it with a meal rich in fiber and protein. This balance ensures that your gut receives nutrients while you enjoy your favorite foods. Creating harmony in your diet helps maintain a healthy microbiome, reducing the risk of digestive issues.

For healthier indulgence options, there are many ways to satisfy cravings while supporting your gut. Dark chocolate, for instance, is a delightful alternative to milk chocolate. It has less sugar and is rich in antioxidants, making it a more gut-friendly choice. Homemade baked goods with natural sweeteners like maple syrup or honey can satisfy your sweet tooth. These natural options are less processed and often contain additional nutrients that benefit your health. By choosing wisely, you can enjoy the pleasures of indulgence without derailing your health goals.

Let me share a story about my friend, Sam, who has mastered balancing indulgence with maintaining gut health. Sam loves pizza and used to indulge without much thought, which often led to discomfort. Now, he designates Fridays as his "pizza day," enjoying a slice or two with a salad. This approach allows him to enjoy his favorite food as part of a balanced meal. Another friend, Lisa, incorporates "cheat meals" into her routine, allowing herself one indulgent meal weekly. She finds that these planned indulgences help her stay on track the rest of the time, preventing feelings of restriction. These stories highlight that you can relish indulgence while keeping your gut happy with some planning.

Finding the best balance between indulgence and health is a

personal journey. It is about understanding your body and what makes you feel good. By allowing yourself the occasional treat, you create a sustainable approach to health that celebrates food in all its forms. This perspective benefits your gut and enriches your overall well-being, reminding you that life is to be enjoyed, one delicious bite at a time.

GUT HEALTH FOR ACTIVE LIFESTYLES

Whether you are a weekend warrior or a competitive athlete, your gut health plays a crucial role in athletic performance and recovery. The connection between physical activity and digestive wellness works both ways—exercise can improve your gut health, while a healthy gut supports better athletic performance. Understanding this relationship helps you optimize your training and prevent common digestive issues from interfering with your fitness goals. As you increase your activity level, your gut needs specific support to handle exercise demands while maintaining optimal function.

Exercise and the Microbiome

Physical activity profoundly changes the gut microbiome, often leading to greater bacterial diversity and improved metabolic function. Regular exercise increases the abundance of beneficial bacteria that produce SCFA, which helps reduce inflammation and support energy metabolism. These changes can vastly improve the body's ability to process nutrients and maintain stable blood sugar levels during workouts. Even moderate exercise, when done consistently, can lead to positive adaptations in gut bacteria composition.

However, intense exercise can temporarily stress your digestive system, particularly during long or high-intensity sessions. Blood flow shifts away from your digestive organs to support working muscles, leading to temporary changes in gut function. This "exercise-induced gut permeability" might cause discomfort or digestive issues during or after workouts. Understanding these effects helps you prepare for and minimize potential digestive disruptions while maintaining your training schedule.

Sports Nutrition for Gut Health

The foods you choose to fuel your workouts significantly impact your performance and gut health. Athletes need more calories and nutrients to support their activity level, but these increased demands must be met while maintaining digestive comfort. Focus on easily digestible carbohydrates before workouts, such as ripe bananas or white rice, which provide energy without overwhelming your digestive system. Including adequate protein throughout the day supports muscle recovery while providing the building blocks for digestive enzyme production.

Timing your nutrition becomes particularly important when considering gut health in sports. Eating too close to your exercise times can lead to digestive distress, while not eating enough can impact performance. Creating a personalized fueling strategy that considers both the timing and composition of meals helps optimize athletic performance and digestive comfort. This might mean experimenting with different pre-workout meals and snacks to discover what works best for your body and training schedule.

Pre- and Post-Workout Gut Support

Proper meal timing and composition are key to supporting your gut before exercise. A pre-workout meal should be consumed two to four hours before training, allowing time for proper digestion. This meal should be relatively low in fat and fiber to prevent digestive discomfort during exercise. Some athletes benefit from simple carbohydrate sources like sports drinks or energy gels during longer sessions. However, these should be tested during training, not during race day or important events.

Post-workout nutrition has a crucial role in recovery and gut health maintenance. The recovery window after exercise presents an opportunity to replenish nutrients and support gut repair. Including easily digestible protein sources helps repair exercise-induced gut damage while supporting muscle recovery. Anti-inflammatory foods like tart cherries or turmeric can help manage exercise-induced inflammation, which affects both muscles and the digestive system.

Beyond essential nutrition, specific gut-support strategies can enhance your athletic experience. Probiotics designed for athletes have shown promise in reducing exercise-induced gut permeability and supporting immune function during heavy training. Staying well-hydrated before, during, and after exercise is vital. Again, it helps maintain proper digestive function and promotes overall performance. Some athletes find that specific supplements like L-glutamine or collagen peptides help maintain gut barrier integrity during intense training.

The key to maintaining gut health while pursuing athletic goals is balancing supporting performance and protecting digestive function. This often requires experimentation and careful attention to how your body responds to different nutrition strategies. Working with sports nutrition professionals who understand performance needs and gut health can help you develop an individualized plan that supports your athletic goals while maintaining digestive wellness. Remember that as your training evolves, your gut health needs may change, requiring periodic nutrition and supplementation strategy adjustments.

This chapter explored how dietary choices impact gut health, from the benefits of whole foods to the joys of mindful indulgence. The next chapter examines how supplements can further support a healthy gut, providing additional tools to enhance wellness.

CHAPTER 6

SUPPLEMENTS AND THEIR ROLE

When I first stepped into the world of gut health, I was greeted by many options in the supplement aisle. The shelves were filled with promises of improved digestion and vitality. Determining the right probiotic supplement can be overwhelming. However, with the correct guidance, you can make an informed decision that suits your needs. Probiotics, often hailed as beneficial bacteria, are not a magic solution but a supportive tool in the journey to a healthy gut. They are vital in balancing the gut microbiome, supporting digestion, and most importantly, overall wellness. However, not all probiotic supplements are the same, and understanding what makes one effective is essential to reaping their benefits. This understanding will reassure you that you are on the right path to better gut health and overall well-being.

AN INTRODUCTION TO PROBIOTIC SUPPLEMENTS

An effective probiotic supplement is like a well-composed symphony, requiring the right combination of strains and strength to perform harmoniously. One key factor is the presence of multiple bacterial strains. Diversity is important because different strains offer unique benefits, like how various instruments contribute to a more decadent musical piece. According to a study, probiotic products with diverse bacterial strains exhibit the best antibacterial activity against common gastrointestinal pathogens. Therefore, when selecting a probiotic, consider multi-strain options that enhance your gut's ability to fend off harmful bacteria. Also, consider the colony-forming units (CFUs). These indicate the number of viable bacteria in the supplement. A higher CFU count can mean a more potent probiotic, but it is not always the best choice. The effectiveness of probiotics also depends on the strains included and their specific functions.

Understanding the specific health benefits of probiotic strains is crucial when choosing the right supplement. This knowledge empowers you to tailor your probiotic intake to your health objectives, ensuring you get the most out of your supplement. For instance, lactobacillus rhamnosus is often recommended for digestive health, as it aids in reducing symptoms of IBS and supports overall gut function. If you focus on boosting your immune system, bifidobacterium lactis might be the strain for you, as it is known for enhancing immune response and maintaining gut barrier integrity. This understanding allows you to make informed choices about your health, promoting a sense of control and confidence in your gut health journey.

Timing and method are key to maximizing the benefits of probiotics. Probiotics can enhance absorption and ensure the bacteria survive the stomach's acidic environment. Meals act as a buffer, helping probiotics reach the intestines where they do their work. Consistency is also essential. Incorporating probiotics into your daily routine supports sustained effects, as regular intake helps maintain a balanced gut microbiome. Think of it as nurturing a garden; regular watering keeps the plants thriving. Similarly, consistent probiotic intake keeps your gut flora flourishing, promoting a healthy digestive ecosystem.

Misconceptions about probiotics abound, so it is vital to set the record straight. One common myth is that all probiotics require refrigeration. While some do, many modern formulations are shelf-stable, using advanced packaging techniques like nitrogen flushing or blister packs to ensure bacteria viability. Always check the label for storage instructions. Another misconception is that more CFUs equate to better results. This is not necessarily true, as the effectiveness of a probiotic depends on the strains and how well they address your specific health needs. It is about quality and targeted action, not just quantity. It is also important to note that while probiotics are generally safe, they may cause mild side effects like gas or bloating in some individuals, particularly when first taking them. If you experience any persistent or severe side effects, it is best to consult a healthcare professional.

Interactive Element: Probiotic Selection Checklist

To help you navigate the probiotic selection process, here is a simple checklist:

1. **Identify Your Health Goal**: Digestive health, immunity, or both?
2. **Check for Multi-Strain Options**: Look for diversity to support various functions.
3. **Evaluate CFUs**: Consider the appropriate strength for your needs.
4. **Match Strains to Concerns**: Choose strains like lactobacillus rhamnosus for gut health or bifidobacterium lactis for immunity.
5. **Review Storage Instructions**: Ensure the supplement's storage aligns with your lifestyle.
6. **Be Consistent**: Plan to take your probiotic daily with meals for optimal absorption.

Using this checklist, you can confidently pick a probiotic supplement that aligns with your wellness goals.

PREBIOTIC VS. PROBIOTIC SUPPLEMENTS: WHAT IS THE DIFFERENCE?

We covered this briefly in the first chapter, but let us now look at the critical differences between prebiotics and probiotics in the context of supplements. Navigating the world of gut health supplements might seem complex, but understanding prebiotics and probiotics is key to making informed choices. Think of your gut like a garden: probiotics are the beneficial organisms you plant, while prebiotic supplements are the specialized fertilizer that helps them thrive. Probiotic supplements typically contain specific strains like lactobacillus and bifidobacterium, available in capsules, powders, or liquid forms. Prebiotic supplements, often containing ingredients like inulin, FOS (fructooligosaccharides), or GOS (galactooligosaccharides), work behind the scenes to feed these beneficial bacteria.

When choosing supplements, consider starting with a high-quality probiotic that offers multiple strains and adequate CFUs, typically between 1 and 50 billion, depending on your needs. Look for prebiotics containing well-researched fibers, and consider combination supplements that offer prebiotics and probiotics (synbiotics) for a comprehensive approach (more on this later). Just remember that timing matters with supplements. Take probiotics on an empty stomach for optimal absorption, and space out prebiotic supplements throughout the day to avoid digestive discomfort. Also, keep your probiotic supplements away from hot beverages, as heat can deactivate the beneficial bacteria.

DIGESTIVE ENZYMES: AIDING YOUR GUT'S NATURAL PROCESSES

Imagine your digestive system as a bustling factory, where food is the raw material that needs to be broken down into usable products. This is where digestive enzymes come into play, acting as the hardworking employees that facilitate the breakdown of food into nutrients your body can absorb. Each type of enzyme has a specific role in processing different macronutrients. Protease breaks down proteins into amino acids essential for muscle repair and growth. Lipase targets fats, converting them into fatty acids and glycerol, which your body can use for energy and cell structure. On the other hand, amylase handles carbohydrates, breaking them down into simple sugars like glucose, fueling your cells with energy. Without these enzymes, your body would struggle to extract essential nutrients from your foods, leading to symptoms like indigestion and bloating.

You might wonder how to recognize when your body is not producing enough vital enzymes. Persistent bloating after meals is a common sign. If you experience discomfort or feel unusually full, even after eating a small amount, it could indicate that your food is not being broken down efficiently. Similarly, if you have difficulty digesting specific foods like dairy or gluten, it might be due to a lack of the enzymes needed to process these substances. Lactase, for instance, is an enzyme required to break down dairy products' sugar (lactose). Without enough lactase, you might experience bloating, gas, or diarrhea after consuming dairy. Determining these signs can be the first step toward addressing digestive enzyme deficiencies and improving your gut health.

Choosing the right digestive enzyme supplement can help alleviate these symptoms and support your body's natural processes. When selecting a supplement, look for broad-spectrum enzyme blends. These products contain a variety of enzymes, each targeting different macronutrients, ensuring comprehensive digestive support. It is like hiring a team of specialists with expertise to tackle every aspect of digestion. Checking the label for enzyme activity levels is also essential. This information tells you how effectively the enzymes will perform their tasks. Higher activity levels often indicate a more potent supplement capable of efficiently breaking down food. However, remember that more is not always better; the key is finding a balanced product that meets your dietary needs.

Quick Reference: Common Digestive Enzymes

Consider referring to the list below, which outlines common digestive enzymes and their functions:

- **Protease**: Breaks down proteins into amino acids.
- **Lipase**: Transforms fats into fatty acids and glycerol.
- **Amylase**: Processes carbohydrates into simple sugars.
- **Lactase**: Breaks down lactose in dairy.
- **Cellulase**: Helps digest cellulose in plant cell walls.

This list can be a handy reference when selecting a supplement. It will help you understand which enzymes are included and their benefits.

Adding enzyme supplements to your daily health regimen can bolster your digestive system's efficiency, which is particularly beneficial for those who regularly encounter discomfort following meals. These supplements assist in the meticulous breakdown of food, facilitating a smoother digestive process that can significantly diminish bloating and enhance nutrient absorption. As you navigate the array of enzyme supplements available, engaging with a healthcare provider for tailored guidance is crucial. This step ensures that your selected supplement complements your dietary needs and aligns with your wellness objectives. A healthcare professional can offer insights based on your health history and current conditions, helping you make an informed choice that optimizes your digestive health.

SYNBIOTICS: THE POWER OF COMBINED FORCES

Think of synbiotics as the ultimate team effort in gut health. As mentioned, these supplements blend the benefits of prebiotics and probiotics, creating a dynamic duo that works together to promote a healthy gut. As discussed, prebiotics are non-digestible fibers and act as food for probiotics (beneficial bacteria). When you combine them, prebiotics enhance the survival and growth of probiotics, ensuring they thrive in your gut. This powerful combination supports a balanced and diverse microbiome, vital for maintaining digestive health. By providing a nurturing environment for probiotics, synbiotics help fortify your gut, making it more resilient against imbalances and disruptions. It is like having a personal trainer and nutritionist rolled into one, each playing their part to keep your gut in peak condition.

The benefits of synbiotic supplements go beyond what prebiotics and probiotics can achieve separately. When used in tandem, they improve the efficacy of restoring gut balance, making it more efficient. This enhanced support not only aids digestion but also bolsters immune health, as a well-balanced gut plays a crucial role in protecting against pathogens. Imagine it as a comprehensive wellness plan for your gut, simultaneously addressing multiple aspects of health. Synbiotics provide a holistic approach, ensuring that your gut receives both the bacteria it needs and the food to sustain them. This synergy offers a robust defense against digestive issues and immune challenges, promoting overall well-being.

Incorporating synbiotics into your diet can be as simple as selecting the right foods or supplements. For example, yogurt with added inulin fiber is a delicious way to enjoy a synbiotic snack. The probiotics in yogurt are supported by inulin, a prebiotic that helps them thrive.

Note that inulin is a naturally occurring soluble prebiotic fiber from the fructan family, found abundantly in chicory root, Jerusalem artichoke, garlic, onions, bananas, asparagus, and leeks. This beneficial fiber plays a crucial role in digestive health by providing beneficial gut bacteria and promoting regular bowel movements while supporting calcium absorption and blood sugar regulation. Inulin supplements offer numerous health benefits, but it is essential to introduce them gradually into your diet, as consuming too much too quickly can lead to digestive discomfort, bloating, and gas. Most people can tolerate between five to ten grams daily, though those following a low-FODMAP diet may need to limit or avoid inulin-rich foods.

Another option is synbiotic capsules, which contain specific strains of probiotics along with prebiotic fibers. These supplements are designed to deliver both benefits conveniently, making it easy to support gut health daily. By including synbiotic foods or supplements in your routine, you can give your gut the full support it needs to function optimally.

To optimize synbiotics' benefits, it is crucial to integrate them into your daily health regimen with precision and care. Consuming them alongside meals can significantly boost their absorption. This strategic timing allows the prebiotics and probiotics to synchronize effectively, enhancing their collaborative impact on gut health. Emphasizing consistency in their use is paramount for achieving lasting benefits. A regular, disciplined intake fosters a stable and harmonious gut microbiome, laying the groundwork for a robust digestive system.

Envision this practice as a daily nurturing ritual for your gut, supplying it with a well-rounded diet of essential nutrients and beneficial bacteria it needs to flourish. Adopting synbiotics as a core component of your daily health routine establishes a solid foundation for enduring gut wellness. This commitment to gut health empowers you to experience the full spectrum of advantages from a balanced and resilient digestive system, including improved digestion, enhanced immune function, and overall well-being.

NAVIGATING THE SUPPLEMENT AISLE: TRUSTWORTHY BRANDS

Walking into the supplement aisle can feel like stepping into a maze. The choices can be overwhelming, with each brand claiming to be the best. Choosing reputable brands is crucial when it comes to supplements. A trustworthy company will ensure that its products are both safe and effective. Find brands that have third-party testing and certification. This tells you that an independent organization has verified the supplement's quality and safety. Certifications from organizations like NSF (National Sanitation Foundation) International or ConsumerLab.com provide an extra layer of security, confirming that what is on the label is in the bottle. These certifications are like a seal of trust, ensuring you buy a product that delivers on its promises.

Transparency is another key factor in choosing supplements. A reputable brand will provide transparent ingredient sourcing and manufacturing processes. This means they are upfront about where they get their ingredients and how they make their products. Transparency builds trust between you and the company, showing they have nothing to hide. When evaluating supplement quality, clear labeling is a must. Check for a comprehensive ingredient list, ensuring you know exactly what you consume. Brands that back their claims with research or studies demonstrate their commitment to evidence-based products. This approach reassures you that scientific support for the product's benefits enhances your confidence in its efficacy.

Navigating the marketing claims on supplement packaging can be tricky. Keep an eye out for red flags like "miracle cure" language. These are often exaggerated claims that promise unrealistic results. Be skeptical of health claims that sound too good to be true. A healthy dose of skepticism can prevent you from falling for marketing gimmicks. Supplements are meant to support your health, not serve as a cure-all. Understanding this helps you make educated decisions in the supplement aisle.

Reliable resources are invaluable for your research. Again,

websites like ConsumerLab.com and NSF International offer unbiased supplement reviews and testing results, providing insights into which products meet high quality and safety standards. Consulting healthcare professionals is also a wise step. They can offer individualized instruction based on your specific health needs, guiding you toward the right supplements. Their expertise can help you untangle the complexities of supplement selection, ensuring you choose wisely.

With careful consideration, you can confidently choose supplements that support your health goals. Making informed decisions involves understanding what to look for in a reputable brand, recognizing red flags, and utilizing reliable resources. This approach enhances your health journey and empowers you to take charge of your wellness. As we conclude this chapter on supplements, remember that making smart choices today can pave the way for a healthier tomorrow.

CHAPTER 7

OVERCOMING COMMON CHALLENGES

Remember the last time you meticulously planned a week's worth of healthy meals, only to have life throw curveballs at you, leaving your good intentions scattered like leaves in the wind? You are not alone. Our busy lives often challenge our ability to stick to gut-friendly habits. Juggling work commitments, family responsibilities, and social engagements can make it seem impossible to prioritize health. It is easy to let your well-being slide to the back burner when you are constantly on the go. But maintaining gut health does not have to be an all-or-nothing endeavor. Even amid the chaos, small, strategic changes can help you stay on track and empower you to take control of your health. When consistently applied, these changes can significantly affect your gut health.

Staying on Track with Meal Preparation and Health

Let us start with meal preparation, a key strategy for anyone with a packed schedule. The idea is simple: devote a few hours once a week to prepare meals that can last several days. This might sound daunting, but consider it a gift to your future self. Imagine opening the fridge after a hectic day to find a ready-made, nutritious meal waiting for you. By preparing meals in bulk, you reduce the daily stress of determining what to eat, ensuring that your choices support your gut health. This convenience can be a relief amid a busy week. Think about using an instant pot or slow cooker, which can be lifesavers in the kitchen. They allow you to cook hearty, gut-friendly meals with minimal effort and supervision. Throw in some vegetables, lean proteins, and spices in the morning. By supper time, you will have a delicious meal ready to enjoy.

As I mentioned, meal-planning apps are another efficient method to save time while eating healthy. These digital tools can streamline grocery shopping by organizing your list and suggesting recipes based on your dietary preferences. With a well-organized plan, you can shop more efficiently, ensuring you have all the ingredients needed for your prepped meals. This saves time and reduces the temptation to veer off course with convenience foods. Setting reminders for hydration and mindful eating breaks can also help you stay on track. These small nudges throughout the day encourage you to take a moment for your health, whether sipping water regularly or pausing to enjoy your meals without distractions.

Incorporating health into your daily routine does not require drastic changes. It is about finding moments to introduce small habits that collectively make a difference. Short walks during lunch breaks, for instance, can help you stay active and invigorate your mind and body. These brief moments of movement can also aid digestion and boost your mood, making them a valuable addition to your day. When snacking, opt for quick, healthy options like nuts or fruit. These snacks are easy to pack and can be lifesaving during busy days when hunger strikes. They provide essential nutrients without derailing your gut health goals.

Time management is crucial here. Tools like planners or digital calendars can help you allocate time for meal prep and physical activity. Marking these activities as non-negotiables in your schedule ensures they become a consistent part of your routine. By prioritizing these small yet impactful habits, you can maintain your gut health without feeling overwhelmed by life's demands.

Reflection Section: Scheduling Your Health

Reflect deeply on the rhythm of your typical day. Pinpoint those moments ripe for incorporating gut-health-enhancing practices. A transformative approach to consider is dedicating a slice of your weekend—perhaps a Sunday afternoon—exclusively to meal preparation. Investing just a handful of hours into cooking and safely storing away a variety of nutrient-dense meals can arm you with the tools for a triumphant, health-focused week ahead. This is not merely about having meals ready but about empowering yourself to make gut-nourishing choices without the daily hassle.

Moreover, scrutinize your daily agenda for brief interludes that are often overlooked and can be optimized for a health boost. For instance, a mere fifteen-minute break after lunch can be ideal for a brisk walk. This simple activity stimulates digestion and recharges your mental energy. Use these insights to tailor a comprehensive action plan that embeds gut-health-promoting practices into the fabric of your daily life. Stress the importance of setting realistic, attainable goals. It is about integrating these habits consistently rather than reaching for perfection from day one. This approach can be encouraging and motivating, making your health journey feel more achievable. Remember, the small, consistent steps lead to significant progress in your gut health.

Documenting each step of this journey, however small it may seem, is vital for gauging your progress. Every conscious choice, whether opting for a snack that nurtures your gut or committing to a brief exercise, marks a significant stride toward enhanced gut health. Embrace and celebrate each milestone achieved on this path. Recognizing your effort in making healthier choices reaffirms your dedication and fuels your motivation to persist. These seemingly modest victories lay the groundwork for a solid foundation of gut well-being and overall health, propelling you forward on your journey to a more balanced and vibrant life.

MANAGING SOCIAL SITUATIONS WHILE ON A GUT-HEALTH PLAN

Imagine you are at a lively dinner party, surrounded by friends. The table is filled with tempting dishes, and the air buzzes with laughter. Yet, there is a nagging thought in your mind: *How can I stick to my gut health goals amid the social pressure to indulge?* It is a common dilemma. Social gatherings often present challenges like peer pressure to indulge in foods that do not align with your health objectives and a lack of healthier options. You might find yourself at a buffet with limited choices, wondering how to navigate these situations without compromising your goals.

One of the most practical strategies for social gatherings is to bring a healthy dish to share. This guarantees you have something suitable to eat and introduces others to nutritious options. Think of it as a way to contribute to the meal while staying true to your dietary needs. If bringing a dish is impossible, consider eating a small meal beforehand. Filling up on nutrient-dense foods at home can curtail your hunger and make it easier to resist unhealthy temptations. This simple step enables you to make better choices when faced with a spread of less-than-ideal options.

Communication with friends and family is another key component of staying on track. Let your loved ones know about your gut health goals and dietary needs. Explain why certain foods might not be the best for you, and invite them to join you in health-conscious activities. Whether suggesting a hike and healthy picnic lunch instead of a lavish brunch or hosting a potluck focusing on wholesome dishes, involving others in your healthy lifestyle can foster understanding and support; you will likely find those close to you more willing to accommodate your needs than expected. Plus, sharing your journey can inspire others to prioritize their health.

It is important to remember that balance and flexibility are crucial in maintaining a sustainable lifestyle. Occasional indulgences are acceptable and can be a healthy part of your routine. Let yourself enjoy a slice of cake at a birthday party or a special dish at a family gathering. The key is to savor these moments mindfully, without guilt, and to focus on maintaining healthy habits in the long run. Life is about enjoying the little moments; food is often a central part of celebrations. Focusing on balance allows you to enjoy these occasions without feeling like you have derailed your progress.

Interactive Element: Reflection Exercise

Reflect on a recent social event that challenged your gut health commitments. Identify the hurdles you encountered in maintaining your dietary plan, consider the strategies you employed to navigate these obstacles, and think about what you might do differently in the future:

- Was it the limited selection of gut-friendly foods, the temptation from less healthy options, or perhaps the social pressure to partake in everything on offer that presented as problems?
- Did you plan to eat before attending, or did you choose to bring a nutritious dish to share?
- Could you have communicated your dietary needs more clearly to your host?

Identifying a go-to healthy option that is easy to prepare and popular with guests could be a solution. Exploring ways to politely decline offers that do not fit your health goals without feeling socially awkward could also help. Take a moment to brainstorm a few actionable strategies that align with your gut-health plan for similar situations. These might include preparing a list of easy, gut-friendly dishes to make and transport, setting up a pre-event eating strategy to avoid hunger, or even practicing a few kind phrases to decline non-compliant foods gracefully.

Document these reflections and strategies. This detailed plan will be a practical guide for navigating social gatherings without compromising your gut health objectives. Keeping this list accessible will remind you that it is entirely possible to partake in the joy of social events while steadfastly adhering to your health goals.

ADDRESSING SLOW PROGRESS: PATIENCE AND PERSISTENCE

Going on a journey to improve gut health can feel like setting sail into the unknown—filled with initial excitement, quickly tempered by the reality of slow progress. This gradual path to wellness is particularly pronounced in gut health, where the fruits of your labor often take time to manifest. Understanding that this journey is more akin to a marathon than a sprint is crucial. Progress may be imperceptible at the outset, but small daily habits lay the groundwork for substantial long-term benefits. It is natural for motivation to wane when immediate results are elusive; however, embracing patience at these moments is essential. The complexity of the gut ecosystem, shaped by diet, lifestyle, stress, and genetic factors, means improvements require time and consistency. Simple measures, such as dietary adjustments and the strategic use of probiotics, contribute incrementally to your overall health. These initial changes might not yield immediate visible outcomes, but deep within your gut, a transformation is underway.

The timeline for noticeable improvements in symptoms like digestion and energy levels varies significantly among individuals. It may span weeks or even months, underscoring the importance of dedication and allowing your body the necessary time to adapt to these positive shifts. Maintaining motivation throughout this slow transformation is paramount. A highly effective strategy to stay encouraged, and one I have been constantly touting, is keeping a health journal. Documenting your journey, from the subtle shifts to the more pronounced changes, can uplift your spirits. For instance, noting an uptick in energy following the introduction of a gut-friendly breakfast can serve as a powerful motivator. Celebrating these victories, regardless of size, fosters a sense of achievement and sharpens your focus on the goals ahead. Each positive change, recognized and recorded, becomes a milestone on your path to better health.

The experience of Bill, who dealt with persistent bloating for years, illustrates the virtue of persistence. Initially skeptical about the benefits of dietary adjustments, Bill decided to experiment by slowly integrating more fiber and fermented foods into his diet. Despite not observing immediate benefits, he remained committed to his new regimen. Over a year, this perseverance paid off, leading to a noticeable reduction in bloating and a significant boost in his energy levels. Bill's narrative underscores the transformative power of patience and steadfastness in overcoming initial hurdles and achieving lasting wellness.

Patience and persistence emerge as invaluable allies in pursuing enhanced gut health. The temptation to seek instant solutions or to discontinue efforts when progress seems to stall is understandable. Yet, it is essential to remember that profound, meaningful change unfolds over time. Focusing on the long-term benefits, like improved digestion, increased energy, and a better mood, can help you embrace the journey with optimism. Recognize that each small step forward is crucial to your broader journey to a healthier, more vibrant you.

DEBUNKING MYTHS AND MISCONCEPTIONS ABOUT GUT HEALTH

Gut health is undeniably a hot topic these days, but with popularity comes a slew of myths and misconceptions that can easily mislead you. One of the most prevalent myths is the idea of quick-fix solutions. Stores are filled with products promising miraculous overnight results for your gut. However, achieving and maintaining gut health is rarely a one-step process. No magic pill can replace the advantages of a balanced diet and lifestyle. Additionally, there is a common oversimplification when it comes to probiotics. Many believe that just any probiotic will do the trick, but in reality, the effectiveness of probiotics can vary greatly depending on the strain and our specific health needs.

Scientific research offers clarity and dispels these myths.

Studies have shown that there is no one-size-fits-all solution for probiotics. Different strains serve different purposes, and their effectiveness can depend on your health condition. For instance, while one strain might support digestive health, another could be more effective for boosting immunity. Furthermore, gut health is a complex interplay of diet, lifestyle, genetics, and more. As we have seen, it is not just about what you eat but how you live. Factors like stress and sleep quality play significant roles in gut health, emphasizing the need for a holistic approach instead of depending solely on dietary changes.

Critical thinking is your best tool to navigate through the noise of misinformation. It is essential to question the health information you come across, especially when it sounds too good to be true. Evaluate sources by checking the credibility of the authors and the evidence supporting their claims. Scientific studies, peer-reviewed articles, and advice from trusted health professionals are the gold standard for reliable information. Consulting with healthcare providers specializing in nutrition or gastroenterology can offer personalized insights and guidance tailored to your unique needs. This approach ensures you make educated decisions based on credible knowledge rather than falling for the marketing hype.

Again, personalization is key when it comes to gut health. What works wonders for one person might not have the same effect on another. This individuality is why cookie-cutter solutions often fall short. Your gut microbiome is as distinct as your fingerprint, influenced by many factors, including diet, environment, and stress levels. As such, it is vital to tailor dietary and lifestyle changes to fit your circumstances and health goals. This might mean experimenting with different foods or supplements to see what best suits your body. Listening to your body and making adjustments based on your feelings can lead to more effective and sustainable health outcomes.

ANTIBIOTICS AND YOUR GUT

While antibiotics are crucial medical interventions for bacterial infections, their impact on gut health extends beyond their intended targets. These medications do not differentiate between harmful pathogens and beneficial bacteria, often leading to significant disruptions in the gut microbiome. Understanding how antibiotics affect the digestive system can help you take practical steps to protect and restore gut health when these medications are necessary. Antibiotic use and gut health represent a delicate balance between effectively treating infections and maintaining microbiome integrity.

Impact on Microbiome

When you take antibiotics, they create what scientists often describe as a "scorched earth" effect in your gut ecosystem. These medications can eliminate vast populations of beneficial bacteria within days, dramatically reducing the diversity and quantity of your gut microbiota. This disruption can lead to immediate effects like diarrhea, bloating, and digestive discomfort. The potential long-term impact is more concerning, as research suggests that some bacterial species may take months or even years to recover if they return.

The loss of beneficial bacteria creates opportunities for less desirable organisms to flourish, potentially leading to an overgrowth of problematic bacteria or fungi. This phenomenon, known as dysbiosis, can manifest in various ways, from digestive issues to immune system challenges. Additionally, antibiotics can affect your body's ability to process and absorb nutrients effectively, as many of these functions rely on a healthy bacterial population. The disruption can also impact the production of essential compounds like SCFA, which play crucial roles in gut health and overall immunity.

Recovery Strategies

Rebuilding gut health after antibiotics requires a strategic approach that supports the restoration of beneficial bacteria while preventing opportunistic infections. Start by introducing probiotic-rich foods like yogurt, kefir, and fermented vegetables into your diet. These foods provide living beneficial bacteria that can help repopulate your gut. However, timing matters—research suggests waiting a few hours between taking antibiotics and consuming probiotics to maximize their effectiveness.

Supporting your gut's recovery also means providing the right environment for beneficial bacteria to thrive. Focus on consuming prebiotic foods that feed helpful bacteria, such as garlic, onions, asparagus, and bananas. Include plenty of fiber-rich foods to provide the necessary building blocks for bacterial growth and diversity. Some people find that specific supplements like L-glutamine or zinc carnosine can help support gut barrier repair during this vulnerable period.

Prevention Protocol

Implementing a prevention protocol when antibiotics are necessary can help minimize their impact on gut health. Before beginning your antibiotic course, take a high-quality probiotic supplement, ideally one that contains multiple strains and many CFUs. Continue this supplementation throughout your antibiotic treatment and for several weeks afterward to support microbiome recovery.

Creating a gut-protective environment before and during antibiotic treatment can help reduce adverse effects. Focus on anti-inflammatory foods and those abundant in antioxidants to support your body's natural healing processes. Consider incorporating specific supplements like saccharomyces boulardii, a beneficial yeast that can help prevent antibiotic-associated diarrhea while remaining unaffected by the antibiotics themselves.

The weeks following antibiotic treatment present a crucial window for supporting gut recovery. During this time, prioritize sleep and stress management, as these factors significantly influence gut healing. Avoid processed foods, excess sugar, and alcohol, which can further disrupt your recovering microbiome. Instead, focus on nutrient-dense, whole foods that support gut health and immune function.

Long-term strategies for protecting your gut from antibiotic damage include building a resilient microbiome through diet and lifestyle choices. Regular consumption of fermented foods, adequate fiber intake, and stress management can help create a more robust gut ecosystem that may resist disruption. Additionally, work with your healthcare provider to ensure antibiotics are only used when necessary, as each course can have cumulative effects on your gut health.

Understanding the broader impact of antibiotics on gut health does not mean avoiding them when medically necessary. Instead, this knowledge empowers you to take protective measures before, during, and after antibiotic treatment. By implementing appropriate recovery strategies and prevention protocols, you can help minimize the disruption to your gut ecosystem while still benefiting from these necessary medications when needed. Remember that recovery is gradual; patience and consistent support for your gut health will yield the best results.

HANDLING SETBACKS: WHAT TO DO WHEN SYMPTOMS PERSIST

Facing setbacks is a natural part of improving your gut health. It is expected to encounter bumps along the way. Remember, these occasional symptoms do not define your progress. They are merely signals from your body, prompting you to reassess and adjust your approach. Sometimes, despite your best efforts, you might find your symptoms lingering. This does not mean you have failed. Instead, it is an opportunity to learn and refine your strategies. Embracing resilience and a positive outlook will help you navigate these challenges, turning temporary setbacks into stepping stones toward lasting health.

A practical approach to addressing persistent symptoms starts by re-evaluating your diet. Even small dietary triggers can have a significant impact on your gut health. As recommended, keep a food diary to track what you eat and how it affects you. This can help you identify intolerances or foods that may exacerbate your symptoms. As outlined, lifestyle factors like stress and sleep quality can influence your gut. Stress can wreak mayhem on your digestive system, while poor sleep can disrupt healing. Remember, prioritizing stress management techniques and ensuring you get enough restful sleep can support your gut health and overall well-being.

Sometimes, your efforts to manage symptoms alone do not yield the desired results. In such cases, seeking professional support is a wise step. Consulting with a gastroenterologist or registered dietitian can provide personalized insights and guidance. These professionals can help determine the principal causes of your symptoms and recommend tailored interventions. They can also offer support with managing complex dietary needs or introduce you to specialized treatments that may be beyond the scope of general advice. Reaching out for help is a proactive approach that can significantly enhance your progress.

Consider Annie's experience. Despite making several dietary changes, she experienced persistent bloating and discomfort. Frustrated but determined, she sought the guidance of a dietitian who worked with her to pinpoint specific food intolerances. With this new information, Annie adjusted her diet and gradually saw an improvement in her symptoms. She also experimented with stress-reducing practices like yoga and meditation, further supporting her gut health. Annie's story illustrates how setbacks can lead to breakthroughs when you remain open to adjusting your approach and seeking help when needed.

Navigating setbacks requires creativity and flexibility. Sometimes, the solution might be something simple you had not considered before. For instance, introducing fermented foods or experimenting with probiotics can help rebalance your gut microbiome. Other times, taking a break from certain foods or activities might be necessary to allow your body to reset. The key is to stay curious and willing to explore different options. By maintaining a mindset focused on learning and growth, you can overcome challenges and continue progressing toward improved gut health.

This chapter has explored the common challenges you might face in improving your gut health. From tackling busy schedules and managing social situations to handling setbacks, each section offers practical strategies to help you stay on track. Progress is not a straight line; setbacks are simply part of the process. You can overcome obstacles and continue toward your wellness goals by staying resilient and open to learning. Next, we will explore the intriguing connection between your gut and mind, exploring how nurturing this relationship can enhance physical and mental well-being.

CHAPTER 8

UNDERSTANDING AND MANAGING STRESS FOR DIGESTIVE HEALTH

I magine waking up to the blare of your alarm clock, your heart pounding, and a sense of unease churning in your stomach. For many, this scenario is familiar. However, understanding that stress does not merely cloud the mind but courses through the body, profoundly influencing gut health, can bring relief. Stress manifests not only as a psychological burden but as a physical force, impacting your physiology, with a focus on the digestive system. This knowledge empowers you, giving you control and confidence to take charge of your gut health. As discussed in previous chapters, our bodies exhibit a vital gut-mind connection. This chapter will examine how stress can impact our gut health and the strategies we can employ to lessen its impact.

THE CONNECTION BETWEEN STRESS AND YOUR GUT

In moments of stress, the body shifts into the primal fight-or-flight mode, signaling the enteric nervous system—the gut's intricate neural network, often dubbed the "second brain." This system, deeply intertwined with the central nervous system, responds to stress by modifying gut motility and secretion, frequently resulting in digestive discomfort. Cortisol, the stress hormone, has a pivotal role by coursing through the body and affecting various functions, from heart rate modulation to digestion disruption. The gut-brain axis represents a dynamic, bidirectional communication channel, a veritable superhighway of signals perpetually exchanged between the brain and the gut. This intricate interaction signifies that while stress can adversely affect your gut, your gut's state can similarly influence your emotional well-being.

Stress exposure can alter the operational pace of your gut, triggering issues such as constipation or diarrhea. The gut microbiota—those trillions of microbes in the digestive tract—emerge as crucial modulators of the body's stress response, impacting your resilience or vulnerability to stress. An imbalance in gut flora can amplify stress reactions, fueling a detrimental loop where stress impairs gut health, which, in turn, exacerbates stress levels. Identifying stress-related gut disturbances requires a keen, detective-like observation of our bodies. Symptoms vary widely, from general bloating and discomfort to more acute conditions like IBS. Stress can heighten gut sensitivity, leading to discomfort and pain post-meal. Notably, digestive irregularities may become more pronounced during intense stress, serving as a corporeal signal that stress is undermining your gut health. Heeding these signs is crucial for maintaining digestive well-being.

This is why it is crucial to counter the impact of stress on the gut by integrating stress-reduction techniques into your daily routine. Deep breathing exercises, yoga, or brief walks can significantly soothe the nervous system. These activities stimulate the parasympathetic nervous system, often celebrated as the "rest-and-digest" state, effectively neutralizing the stress response and fostering healthier digestion. Incorporating these practices need not be daunting; initiating small, manageable steps, such as dedicating five minutes to focused breathing or enjoying a short walk during a lunch break, can positively influence your body's stress management and, by extension, your gut health. These small steps can be encouraging and motivating, showing that even a little effort can make a big difference in your gut health.

Reflection Section: Stress and Your Gut

Pause and reflect on the complex interplay between stress and your body's physiological reactions. Have you noticed a pattern where moments of high stress correlate with episodes of gut discomfort? To delve deeper into this intricate relationship, keeping a detailed journal that chronicles these occurrences is beneficial. In this journal, carefully log every instance of stress, clearly outlining the circumstances and your immediate reactions. Along with these stress events, record any gastrointestinal symptoms, whether bloating, discomfort, alterations in bowel movements, or any other signs of digestive upset.

This systematic approach serves a dual purpose: It illuminates recurring patterns linking stress to gut health issues and identifies specific stressors that significantly impact digestive well-being. Equipped with this valuable insight, you can take informed steps toward making lifestyle adjustments that target these stress-related triggers. Incorporating strategies to manage or mitigate these stressors can profoundly strengthen your overall health, setting you on a path to mastering gut health management with precision and confidence.

MINDFULNESS PRACTICES FOR A HEALTHIER GUT

As I pointed out at the beginning of Chapter 4, sitting down to a meal without distractions, fully present, and savoring each bite is a minimal act of mindfulness that can do wonders for your gut health. Mindfulness focuses on the present moment, which can help lower stress and its harmful effects on your body. When practiced regularly, mindfulness can lead to improved digestion and overall well-being. It encourages you to enjoy your food, making meals more satisfying and nourishing. By reducing stress, mindfulness helps lower cortisol levels and other stress hormones that can wreak turmoil on your gut. This sets the stage for better digestion and nutrient absorption, leaving you feeling more balanced and energized. Emphasizing mindfulness's positive effects can instill hope and optimism in your audience.

Another effective mindfulness technique is the body scan exercise. This involves sitting or lying comfortably and focusing on different body parts, from head to toe. As you focus on each area, notice any sensations or tension without judgment. This practice helps you relax and become more aware of your body's signals, which is particularly beneficial for digestion. By tuning into your body's needs, you can better respond to hunger cues and recognize when you are full.

Mindful breathing is another powerful tool. Taking slow, deep breaths can relax your nervous system, promoting a calm state that aids digestion. Inhale deeply through your nose, then hold for a moment, and exhale slowly through your mouth. This can be especially helpful before meals, setting a peaceful tone for your dining experience.

Incorporating mindfulness into your daily life does not require drastic changes. Begin by putting aside a few minutes each day for mindfulness meditation. Over time, these practices can become a natural part of your routine, offering a moment of calm in a busy day and providing ongoing support for your gut health.

To illustrate the impact of mindfulness, consider the story of Zack, who struggled with IBS for years. He found that stress often triggered his symptoms, leaving him feeling frustrated and uncomfortable. After learning about mindfulness, he decided to give it a try. He began practicing mindful eating and meditation regularly, gradually noticing a reduction in his IBS flare-ups. Zack found that by being more present during meals, he made healthier food choices and felt more in tune with his body's needs. This small change made a big difference in his life, allowing him to enjoy food without fear of discomfort. His experience highlights the potential of mindfulness to improve gut health and enhance well-being. Zack's success story can inspire and motivate your audience to take control of their gut health.

Emotional Eating and Gut Health: Breaking the Cycle

Imagine reaching for a bag of chips after a stressful day, not because you are hungry but because you are searching for comfort. This is emotional eating, where emotions drive your eating habits rather than physical hunger. It is a typical response to stress, boredom, or sadness. However, emotional eating can disrupt gut health, leading to digestive issues and nutrient absorption problems. When you eat in response to emotions, you might choose foods high in sugar and fat, which can upset your digestive system. These foods are deficient in nutrients your body needs, leaving your gut struggling to function at its best. Over time, this pattern can lead to imbalances in your gut microbiota, causing discomfort and long-term health concerns.

Recognizing the triggers of emotional eating is a crucial step in breaking the cycle. Stress, loneliness, or even snacking while watching TV can all prompt emotional eating. One effective way to uncover these patterns is by keeping an emotional eating journal. Track what you eat, when, and how you are feeling at the time. This practice can reveal connections between your emotions and eating habits, highlighting areas where you must make changes. You might notice that you tend to reach for snacks when stressed or eat mindlessly when bored. By knowing these triggers, you can address them in ways that do not involve food.

Overcoming emotional eating requires developing new coping mechanisms. Instead of looking to food for comfort, try engaging in activities that fulfill you emotionally. This might mean calling a friend, taking a walk, or diving into a hobby you love. Again, practicing mindful eating can also help differentiate between true hunger and emotional cravings. Before eating, pause to ask yourself if you are truly hungry or if there is another reason you are reaching for food. This pause can help you make more intentional choices about what and when you eat, supporting your gut health and emotional well-being.

To build healthier eating habits, consider exercises and activities that promote mindful and intentional eating. Start by creating a supportive eating environment. This means setting the table nicely, turning off distractions like your TV or phone, and focusing on your meal. Make eating a dedicated activity rather than a side event. Setting specific, achievable goals for mindful eating can also be beneficial. For instance, spend at least twenty minutes on each meal, focusing on your food's flavors and textures. This encourages you to eat slowly and enjoy your meal, helping your digestion and allowing your body to signal when your stomach is full.

Reflective Exercise: Identifying Emotional Triggers

Initiate a seven-day self-observation journey focused on your eating behaviors and the emotions preceding each meal or snack. Equip yourself with a dedicated notebook or select a notes application on your smartphone. Begin by meticulously documenting the specific times you feel compelled to eat alongside the emotions or situations prompting these impulses. Are these feelings rooted in genuine hunger, or are they manifestations of underlying emotional needs? Detail every item you consume, paying close attention to your emotional state before eating. This introspective exercise aims to unveil the intricate web of emotions entangled with your eating habits. By the week's end, carefully analyze your recorded entries to unearth any recurring patterns or emotional triggers linked to your food choices.

This process of reflection is crucial in illuminating the emotional underpinnings of your eating habits, setting the stage for transformative change. Armed with newfound insights into your emotional eating triggers, you are poised to embark on a mindful eating journey. This awareness empowers you to forge decisions that nourish your body and enhance your emotional well-being and gut health. By consciously addressing these emotional triggers, you can disrupt the cycle of emotional eating, paving the way for a harmonious relationship with food and a thriving gut microbiome.

MEDITATION TECHNIQUES TO SUPPORT DIGESTION

Sometimes, life feels like an endless stream of responsibilities and deadlines, leaving little room for the calmness we crave. What if I told you that meditation could be your secret weapon for supporting digestion and soothing stress-related symptoms? Meditation is more than just a tool for calming the mind; it extends its benefits to your digestive health by promoting and activating the parasympathetic nervous system. This system, often called the "rest-and-digest" mode, helps your body relax and focus on digestion. When you meditate, you invite calmness into your life, which can significantly alleviate stress-induced digestive discomfort. By reducing stress, meditation allows your gut to function more efficiently, enhancing nutrient absorption and reducing inflammation.

You can incorporate various meditation techniques into your routine to support your digestive health. One widespread practice is guided imagery focused on gut relaxation. This technique involves visualizing soothing images, such as a gentle stream or a peaceful forest, which helps your body relax deeply. You can reduce tension and promote a healthier digestive environment by picturing your gut as a calm and balanced space. Progressive muscle relaxation is another effective method. It is when you systematically tense and then release each muscle group. This practice eases physical tension, relieving stress that can affect digestion. Loving-kindness meditation, which fosters positive emotions toward yourself and others, can also affect digestive health. By cultivating feelings of compassion and gratitude, you lower stress and create a positive mindset that supports overall well-being.

Starting a meditation practice does not have to be complicated. Begin by setting a regular meditation schedule that fits your lifestyle. Consistency is key, whether five minutes in the morning or a more extended session before bed. Create a calm and distraction-free space where you can meditate comfortably, whether in a cozy corner of your home or a natural spot. Consider using meditation apps or online resources if you are new to the practice, as they can provide guidance and support. Meditation is a personal journey; finding what works best for you is part of the experience. Be patient with yourself as you explore different techniques and settle into a routine that feels right.

To illustrate the impact of meditation on gut health, let us consider the story of Maria. She had struggled with digestive issues for years, often triggered by stress at work. So, Maria decided to try meditation after hearing about its benefits for both mental and physical health. She began practicing guided imagery and progressive muscle relaxation regularly, finding that these techniques helped her unwind after a long day. Over time, she noticed significantly reduced digestive symptoms, with less bloating and discomfort. Meditation became a cherished part of her routine, offering her a sense of calm and balance that extended beyond her gut. Maria's experience highlights how meditation can be a powerful ally in supporting digestive health, reminding us of the mind-body connection and the importance of nurturing both.

BUILDING EMOTIONAL RESILIENCE FOR BETTER GUT HEALTH

Have you ever noticed how some people bounce back from challenges like rubber bands while others struggle under stress? This ability to recover quickly and adapt to difficult situations is known as emotional resilience, and it has a pivotal role in maintaining gut health. Emotional resilience is a buffer against the stressors that can disrupt your digestive system. When you are resilient, you are better prepared to handle stress without wreaking havoc on your gut. This resilience helps to regulate your body's stress responses, reducing the likelihood of stress-induced gut disturbances. It does not mean you wo not encounter stress, but it enhances your capacity to cope, ensuring that life's inevitable ups and downs do not leave you feeling drained or unwell.

Developing emotional resilience involves cultivating certain traits and skills to fortify your mental and emotional state. One such trait is self-awareness, which allows you to understand your emotional triggers and responses. By recognizing how you react to stress, you can begin to manage it more effectively, preventing it from affecting your gut. Emotional regulation is another key component involving controlling your emotions rather than letting them control you. This skill helps you maintain composure in stressful situations, reducing the physical impact of stress on your body. Positive thinking and adaptability also play a role in resilience. When you approach challenges with an optimistic mindset and a willingness to adapt, you are more likely to navigate stress easily, keeping your gut health intact.

Building emotional resilience is a path that requires intentional effort and practice. Journaling is a powerful tool to process emotions and reflect on experiences. You gain clarity and perspective by jotting down your thoughts and feelings, helping you navigate stress more effectively. Engaging in activities that encourage self-care and well-being is equally important. Whether taking a walk in nature, enjoying a hobby, or simply putting aside time for relaxation, these activities nurture your emotional resilience. They provide a reprieve from stress and a chance to recharge, supporting your mental and physical health.

Another vital aspect of building resilience is connecting with supportive communities. Engaging in support groups focused on mental health can provide a sense of understanding and belonging. These groups provide a safe space to learn from others facing similar challenges and share experiences. Connecting with people through shared interests and activities is also beneficial. Whether it is joining a book club, a sports team, or a local community group, these connections foster resilience by offering social support and encouragement. They remind you that you are not alone in your struggles and that others are there to lend a helping hand.

As we wrap up our exploration of the gut-mind connection, emotional resilience is a cornerstone of gut health. Cultivating resilience protects your gut from the adverse effects of stress and paves the way for better health and well-being. This chapter has shown us how interconnected our mental and physical health are, highlighting the importance of nurturing both. As we move forward, we will explore how these insights can inform our approach to nutrition and lifestyle, offering practical strategies for supporting a healthy gut.

CHAPTER 9

PERSONALIZED GUT-HEALTH PLANS

P icture yourself amid the vibrant energy of a farmers' market on a sunny Saturday morning. The air is filled with the enticing aromas of freshly picked herbs and the earthy scent of produce. You are drawn to the colorful array of vegetables and fruit as you navigate the stalls. Each vendor's stand offers a unique blend of flavor and nutrition, catering to your preferences. This bustling scene is a powerful metaphor for understanding how our bodies communicate their distinct nutritional needs and desires.

Just as you might be drawn to specific fruits and vegetables that tantalize your senses and meet your body's craving for certain nutrients, paying close attention to the subtle cues your body sends enables you to sift through the myriad dietary choices available. This careful listening is crucial on your gut health journey, empowering you to craft a personalized health strategy that aligns with your body's requirements.

By choosing the most beneficial and compatible options from the vast selection life offers, you ensure that your nutritional choices are deeply nourishing and supportive of your health and well-being. This approach to diet, rooted in mindfulness and attentiveness to your body's unique language, paves the way for a profoundly personalized journey toward optimal gut health.

LISTENING TO YOUR BODY: PERSONALIZING YOUR GUT HEALTH JOURNEY

Our bodies constantly communicate with us, offering subtle hints about what they need through hunger cues, energy levels, and mood changes. Recognizing these signals is the first step toward fostering a healthier gut. Think about the last time you felt a genuine hunger pang, not just the urge to snack out of boredom. This awareness is crucial. Tuning into your body's hunger and satiety cues can prevent overeating and help you consume what your body truly needs. Similarly, identifying symptoms linked to specific foods or stressors can be enlightening. Perhaps you have noticed that certain foods make you feel sluggish or stress triggers digestive discomfort. These observations are invaluable in understanding your body's unique responses, empowering you to take control of your health.

Interpreting your body's signals requires some detective work, but it is empowering. As we went over in Chapter 3, distinguishing between food sensitivities and allergies is a good place to start. While a food allergy can cause immediate reactions like hives or swelling, sensitivities often result in subtler symptoms such as bloating or fatigue. Paying attention to changes in your energy levels or mood can also provide insights. A sudden dip in energy after a meal might indicate that your body is not processing certain foods well. Your mood can be another indicator; if you feel irritable or anxious after eating, it might be worth exploring whether your diet plays a role. Understanding these bodily responses allows you to make informed dietary and lifestyle choices tailored to your needs, giving you a sense of control and confidence in your health journey.

Add one mindfulness meditation to your daily routine to enhance your body awareness. This practice encourages you to focus on bodily sensations, making recognizing and interpreting your body's signals easier. During meditation, you may notice how certain areas of your body feel, whether tense or relaxed, and how these sensations change with different thoughts or emotions. Another effective technique is to keep a symptom diary. You can identify patterns over time by jotting down what you eat and how you feel afterward. This practice can reveal connections between specific foods and symptoms, giving you a clearer picture of what works for your body and what does not.

Personalizing your gut health journey is ongoing; a few examples can illustrate its potential impact. One acquaintance, Stephanie, struggled with persistent bloating for years. Meticulous observation and noting her body's responses revealed that dairy was a major trigger. However, by eliminating dairy from her diet, Sophie experienced significant relief from her symptoms, bringing hope and optimism to her health journey. Another individual, Mark, noticed his energy levels plummeted whenever he consumed gluten. He experimented with a gluten-free diet and soon found his energy and focus improved dramatically. These personalized adjustments highlight the power of listening to your body and responding with thoughtful changes, offering hope and optimism for your journey.

Reflection Section: Exploring Your Body's Signals

Reflect on your journey with body awareness. Have you observed how specific foods alter your energy or impact your mood? Starting a symptom diary for at least two weeks can be pivotal in your wellness journey. In this diary, meticulously record every meal, snack, and beverage you consume, alongside any physical sensations or emotional reactions that follow. This practice is not about setting dietary limitations but developing a deep understanding of your body's unique needs and reactions. By paying close attention to your body's hunger signals and the outcomes of mindful eating, you can uncover the foods and habits that truly nourish and satisfy you. This thoughtful engagement with your body's signals enables you to devise a tailored gut-health plan, moving beyond one-size-fits-all advice to create a personalized wellness blueprint.

As you embark on this individualized path, you must perceive your body not as an obstacle but as an ally in your health journey. Your body constantly communicates with you, directing you toward choices that enhance vitality and equilibrium. Embrace this exploratory process with an open heart and patience. The insights you gain regarding your body's likes and dislikes will empower you to make choices that improve your physical well-being and align meaningfully with your lifestyle and health aspirations. Remember, this journey requires patience and understanding, but the rewards are worth it, and you are supported every step of the way.

CREATING A GUT-HEALTH JOURNAL: TRACKING YOUR PROGRESS

As you may have noticed, throughout the book, I have reiterated the benefits of a gut-health journal. It is a valuable tool that allows you to uncover the mysteries of your digestive health and connect the dots between what you eat and how you feel. This is where a gut-health journal comes into play. Maintaining a journal that tracks your dietary habits, symptoms, and overall progress opens the door to increased self-awareness and accountability. It is like having a personal detective that helps you identify correlations between your diet and gut health outcomes. A gut-health journal invites you to become curious about your body, encouraging you to observe and reflect on patterns that might go unnoticed.

Starting your gut-health journal is simpler than you might think. Begin by dedicating a notebook or digital document to this purpose. Structure it in a way that suits you, whether daily entries or weekly summaries. Make it a habit to record every meal, snack, and beverage you consume. Pay attention to the details: note the ingredients, portion sizes, and even the time of day. Alongside your dietary log, document any digestive symptoms you experience, such as bloating, gas, or discomfort. But do not stop there—include notes on your mood and energy levels. These factors are often interconnected, and noticing shifts in your feelings can provide valuable insights into your gut health.

Once you have a few weeks' worth of entries, it is time to play detective and analyze your journal. Review your entries methodically, looking for recurring symptoms or potential triggers. You may notice that certain foods consistently lead to discomfort or that your energy levels dip after specific meals. Recognizing these patterns empowers you to adjust your diet and lifestyle. It is like piecing together a puzzle; each entry adds another layer to your understanding of how your body responds to different foods. Evaluating the impact of dietary changes can also be illuminating. If you have recently introduced a new food or eliminated a potential trigger, consider how these changes affect your symptoms and overall well-being.

Consider the story of Daniel, who struggled with persistent digestive issues for years. Frustrated by the lack of answers from various diets and treatments, he started a gut-health journal. Over the course of months, Daniel noticed a pattern: every time he consumed foods containing soy, he experienced bloating and discomfort. Armed with this knowledge, he eliminated soy from his diet and saw a dramatic improvement in his symptoms. Daniel's case illustrates the transformative power of diligent journaling in identifying and addressing food intolerances. By taking the time to track his dietary habits and symptoms, he could pinpoint a specific trigger and make a meaningful change that enhanced his quality of life.

Interactive Element: Start Your Gut-Health Journal

Start your gut-health journal today! Begin by noting the details of your next meal, including the ingredients and how you feel afterward. Pay attention to any digestive symptoms, mood changes, or fluctuations in energy. Over the next few weeks, continue documenting your meals and observations. Review your entries for patterns or potential triggers as you gather more data. Use this information to experiment with dietary adjustments and see how they impact your gut health. This practice fosters greater self-awareness and empowers you to take control of your well-being.

As you embrace the practice of journaling, remember that this is a tool for exploration and growth, not judgment. It is about attuning to your body's signals and using that knowledge to make educated choices. Your gut-health journal is your roadmap, guiding you toward a deeper understanding of what nourishes and supports you. By consistently tracking your progress, you gain valuable insights that can lead to long-lasting improvements in your digestive health. Through this process, you become an active participant in your wellness journey, equipped with the knowledge to make decisions that align with your needs.

ADJUSTING DIET AND LIFESTYLE FOR INDIVIDUAL NEEDS

As I mentioned, there is no one-size-fits-all approach to optimizing your gut health. Remember, our digestive systems are as unique as fingerprints, so personalized dietary adjustments are crucial. Consider how some individuals might naturally produce more digestive enzymes while others need extra help to break down certain foods. This variability can influence how well you digest and absorb nutrients, ultimately affecting your gut health. Your cultural dietary habits and personal preferences also play significant roles. What works for one person might not work for another, highlighting the importance of tailoring your diet to fit your unique lifestyle and needs.

Making dietary adjustments can seem daunting, but it does not have to be an overwhelming task. Start small and make incremental changes based on your gut health goals. For instance, add some berries to your morning cereal to increase your fiber intake, or opt for whole-grain bread instead of white. Experiment with different cooking styles and ingredients to discover what suits you best. You may find that steaming vegetables makes them easier to digest, or you may enjoy the texture that roasting brings. These minor tweaks can significantly improve your gut health, helping you find a balanced diet that works for you.

As I pointed out before, aside from diet, lifestyle factors like sleep, exercise, and stress management play pivotal roles in gut health. Consistent sleep patterns are essential for gut repair and regeneration. During sleep, your body performs vital maintenance tasks, including healing the gut lining and balancing the microbiome. Try to get seven to nine hours of excellent sleep every night to support these processes. Regular physical activity is another key factor. Exercise enhances gut motility, helping food move efficiently through your digestive tract. Whether it is a workout at the gym, a yoga session, or a brisk walk, staying active can keep your gut functioning optimally. Stress management is equally important. As mentioned, chronic stress can ruin your digestive system, slowing digestion and altering gut flora. Incorporating stress-reduction methods like meditation or deep breathing can significantly affect your gut health and overall well-being.

To illustrate the impact of lifestyle changes on gut health, we can consider Jane, who struggled with sluggish digestion and frequent bloating. She incorporated daily stretching and yoga into her routine to improve her digestion and reduce stress. Over weeks and months, Jane noticed a marked improvement in her digestion, with less bloating and more regular bowel movements. The gentle physical activity and focus on breathing helped her body relax and function more efficiently. This change benefited her gut and improved her mental clarity and mood. Another person, Philip, prioritized getting consistent sleep by establishing a bedtime routine. By going to sleep and waking up at the same time each day, he found that his digestive issues lessened, and he felt more energized throughout the day. These stories highlight how simple lifestyle adjustments can lead to profound improvements in gut health.

Adjusting your diet and lifestyle is a personal journey; it is best to approach it with patience and curiosity. Consider what small changes you can make that align with your goals and preferences. Reflect on your current habits and pinpoint areas where you can make improvements. You could try a new cooking technique or dedicate a few minutes daily to stress-reducing activities. These adjustments do not need to happen all at once; instead, focus on making gradual changes that feel sustainable and enjoyable. By tailoring your approach, you can adopt a personalized plan that supports your gut health and overall well-being.

UNDERSTANDING MICROBIOME TESTING

Microbiome testing has expanded rapidly in recent years, offering new insights into the complex ecosystem living within your gut. While traditional digestive health assessments relied primarily on symptoms and essential lab work, modern testing methods can give a detailed map of your gut bacteria composition. This information can be invaluable in understanding your digestive health, but knowing when and how to use these tests effectively makes all the difference. As technology advances, the ability to peek inside your microbiome becomes more accessible, though interpreting this information requires careful consideration.

Available Testing Options

Several approaches to microbiome testing exist, each offering different insights into gut health. The most common method is stool-based DNA testing, which analyzes the genetic material of bacteria in the digestive tract. These tests can identify bacterial species and their types and quantities, providing a snapshot of microbiome diversity. Some tests go beyond essential identification to examine functional markers, including how well gut bacteria process different nutrients or produce beneficial compounds like SCFA.

More comprehensive testing options might include additional markers such as inflammatory indicators, digestive enzyme levels, and the presence of potential pathogens. Some advanced tests can even assess the metabolic functions of your gut bacteria, providing insights into how well they perform crucial tasks like breaking down fiber or producing vitamins. The choice between basic and comprehensive testing often hinges on your specific health concerns and goals and practical considerations like cost and accessibility.

Interpreting Test Results

Understanding the significance and limitations of microbiome test results is crucial. Your test report might show percentages of different bacterial species, comparing them to reference ranges established from healthy populations. However, what constitutes a "healthy" microbiome can vary significantly between people, and current science is still discovering new aspects of optimal bacterial balance. The key is to interpret these results within the context of your symptoms, health history, and overall wellness goals.

The complexity of microbiome test results often requires professional guidance for proper interpretation. While many testing companies provide essential explanations of their findings, working with a healthcare provider who understands microbiome science can help translate these results into actionable steps. They can help you know which bacterial imbalances might contribute to your symptoms and how to address them through dietary changes, lifestyle modifications, or targeted supplementation.

When to Consider Testing

Several situations might warrant microbiome testing. If you are experiencing persistent digestive symptoms despite dietary changes, testing can help identify underlying imbalances contributing to your discomfort. Those with chronic health conditions affecting digestion or immunity might benefit from understanding their microbiome composition to guide treatment strategies. Additionally, those following specific dietary protocols or taking medications that affect gut health might use testing to monitor the impact of these interventions.

However, testing is not always necessary or beneficial. For many people, focusing on fundamental gut health practices like maintaining a diverse, fiber-rich diet and managing stress might be more valuable than detailed testing. Consider microbiome testing when you have specific health concerns that have not responded to essential interventions or when working with a healthcare provider who can use the results to guide your treatment plan effectively.

The timing of testing also matters. Testing during acute illness or immediately after antibiotics might not accurately represent your typical microbiome state. Similarly, recent dietary changes can temporarily affect your results. Consider testing for the most accurate results when your routine has been relatively stable for several weeks. Some situations warrant repeat testing to track changes, particularly when following a specific treatment protocol or making significant dietary modifications.

The investment in microbiome testing should be weighed against its potential benefits. While these tests can give valuable insights, they are just one part of the larger picture of digestive health. The most beneficial approach often combines testing data with careful attention to symptoms, dietary patterns, and overall health markers. Remember that your microbiome is dynamic and constantly changing in response to diet, lifestyle, and environmental factors. Testing provides a snapshot of this complex system, but maintaining gut health requires ongoing attention to the factors that influence your microbiome daily.

COLLABORATING WITH HEALTHCARE PROVIDERS FOR OPTIMAL RESULTS

Imagine having a team of experts explain optimal gut health. Working with healthcare providers can offer that level of support, providing you with specialized knowledge and access to diagnostic tools that can make a significant difference. When dealing with complex or persistent symptoms, having a professional by your side can help you navigate the intricate landscape of gut health. They bring expertise that might not be available through self-guided efforts, from interpreting test results to recommending targeted treatments. This partnership can be especially beneficial if you face challenges requiring a deeper understanding of your physiological needs.

Choosing the correct healthcare provider is crucial to building a successful support system. It is essential to seek out knowledgeable professionals genuinely interested in gut health. Look for those with expertise in nutrition and gastroenterology, as they often have the most relevant training and experience. But do not stop there. Consider practitioners who adopt a holistic and integrative approach, valuing the connection between diet, lifestyle, and overall health. This means they should be open to discussing various aspects of your life that might impact your gut, from stress levels to sleep patterns. A supportive provider will work with you to create a plan that aligns with your health goals and respects your preferences.

Effective communication with your healthcare worker is essential to achieving personalized goals. Before appointments, take the time to prepare questions and concerns. Think about what you have noticed in your body and what you hope to achieve. This preparation ensures that you make the most of your time together, allowing you to address the issues that matter most. Sharing your gut-health journal entries can be incredibly valuable, providing concrete data to inform your discussions. These entries offer insights into your dietary habits, symptoms, and progress, helping your provider better understand your situation. Open and honest communication develops a collaborative relationship, empowering you to partake actively in your health journey.

To illustrate the power of these partnerships, consider the story of Anastasia, who struggled with severe digestive issues for years.

Despite trying various diets and supplements, her symptoms persisted, leaving her frustrated and exhausted. She sought professional guidance and found a nutritionist and gastroenterologist who worked together to develop a comprehensive plan for her. Through a blend of dietary changes, targeted supplements, and stress management techniques, Anastasia began to notice improvements. Her bloating decreased, her energy levels rose, and she felt more in control of her health. The support and expertise of her healthcare team played a pivotal role in her progress, highlighting the impact of professional collaboration.

Another example is David, who faced chronic gut discomfort that interfered with his daily life. He contacted a healthcare provider specializing in gut health and worked with them to identify potential triggers through testing and observation. With their guidance, David discovered that wheat and dairy were exacerbating his symptoms. He achieved significant relief by eliminating these from his diet and gradually reintroducing other beneficial foods. His provider's expertise and personalized approach were instrumental in his journey to improved health, demonstrating the value of professional support in navigating complex gut issues.

These stories show that collaboration with healthcare providers is not just about receiving instructions. It is about building a partnership based on mutual respect and shared goals. Your provider becomes an ally, offering insights and guidance while empowering you to take charge of your health. As you explore this path, remember that you have the right to choose a provider who resonates with you, listens to you, and values your input. The right partnership can make a difference in your gut health journey, providing the tools and support you need for lasting success. In the next chapter, we will explore long-term strategies for maintaining the gut health improvements you have made, ensuring that your progress continues to thrive.

CHAPTER 10

LONG-TERM GUT HEALTH STRATEGIES

Imagine waking up refreshed, feeling like you have had the best night's sleep, with your energy levels so high that you could take on the world. You head to the kitchen, and instead of reaching for sugary cereals or processed snacks, you instinctively choose foods that nourish your body and your gut. This is not just a fantasy—it is the reality of embracing lifestyle changes focused on long-term gut health. The key to this transformation lies not in quick fixes but in adopting consistent, maintainable practices that become second nature over time.

TAKING SMALL STEPS TOWARD GUT HEALTH

One of the most potent aspects of achieving lasting gut health is prioritizing gradual adjustments over drastic changes. Quick fixes might promise immediate results but rarely stand the test of time. Instead, focus on developing routines that naturally incorporate gut-friendly habits. Start small, like adding fiber-rich vegetables such as broccoli or spinach to your dinner, buying whole grains like brown rice or quinoa over processed ones, or incorporating fermented foods like yogurt or kimchi into your diet. These incremental changes, though simple, can profoundly affect your digestive system and overall well-being. By consistently making these choices, you set the foundation for long-term health.

As we discussed, an essential area of focus for maintaining gut health is ensuring you get consistent sleep. Sleep is when your body submits to repair and rejuvenation, including your gut. Again, aim for a regular sleep pattern, ideally seven to eight hours a night. This helps sustain a healthy balance in your gut microbiota and supports digestion. Lack of sleep can disrupt your gut flora, leading to problems like inflammation and impaired digestion. So, consider your bedtime routine sacred. Wind down with activities that relax you, like reading or meditating. These habits improve sleep quality and enhance your gut's ability to repair itself.

Regular physical activity is another cornerstone of supporting gut motility. Exercise stimulates your intestinal muscles' natural contractions, promoting effective digestion and reducing the risk of constipation. Any movement, whether a brisk walk, a yoga session, or a more intense workout, is beneficial. Aim for at least thirty minutes of moderate-intensity exercise most days of the week. It burns calories and keeps your digestive system in motion. Plus, exercise is a fantastic stress reliever, a bonus for your gut and mind.

Making lifestyle changes stick can be challenging, but there are strategies to help ensure your success. Start by setting realistic and achievable goals. Instead of aiming for an overnight overhaul, focus on one change at a time. You might drink more water daily or swap soda for herbal tea. Use habit-tracking tools to monitor your progress. Apps and journals can be great for this, visually representing your commitment and achievements. Seeing your progress can motivate you, especially on more challenging days when old habits try to creep back in.

Interactive Element: Habit Tracker

Create a simple habit tracker. Draw a grid with days of the week across the top and your new habits down the side. Check off each habit as you complete it daily. At the end of the week, review your progress and celebrate your achievements, no matter how small.

Let us look at some real-life success stories for some inspiration. Consider Sarah, a busy professional who struggled with digestive issues for years due to her hectic lifestyle. She decided to make small changes, starting with her breakfast routine. She swapped sugary cereals for oatmeal topped with fruits and nuts, a quick and nutritious option for her busy mornings. Gradually, she added more fiber-rich foods and prioritized daily walks during her lunch break. Over time, Sarah noticed a massive improvement in her digestion and energy levels, which helped her better manage her work and personal life. Then there is Timothy, a student who realized his late-night snacking affected his sleep and gut health. He committed to a consistent bedtime, cut back on heavy evening meals, and introduced a relaxing pre-sleep routine. The results? Better sleep and a happier gut. These stories show that sustainable changes, while taking time, can lead to lasting health benefits, no matter your lifestyle.

The path to long-term gut health is paved with small, consistent steps. You can reach a healthier, more balanced life by embracing gradual changes, focusing on key lifestyle areas, and employing strategies to make these changes stick—your gut and so your future self will thank you.

Building a Supportive Gut Health Community

Imagine setting out on a mission to improve your gut health only to discover you are not alone. Many others are on similar paths, and connecting with them can transform your experience. Engaging with a supportive community does more than provide company—it amplifies your motivation. It gives many tips and insights to make your gut health goals more achievable. Picture this: sharing your struggles with someone who understands or swapping recipes that make integrating fiber into your diet feel less like a chore and more like a shared adventure. This sense of solidarity can be a huge motivator, propelling you forward even when challenges arise and making you feel supported and less alone.

The digital age makes finding or forming a gut health community more effortless than ever. Social media and online groups devoted to gut wellness offer platforms to ask questions, share experiences, and learn from others' journeys. These virtual spaces are teeming with individuals eager to share what has worked for them and learn from your experiences. Look for groups that resonate with your interests, whether fermentation enthusiasts, those tackling specific digestive issues, or general gut health support. Beyond the virtual world, consider local meetups or workshops focused on health and wellness. These gatherings provide a more personal touch, allowing face-to-face interactions and the opportunity to build lasting connections with people who share your health priorities.

Being part of a community is not just about taking but also about giving. Your experiences, whether triumphs or setbacks, can offer invaluable insights to others. Share your progress and challenges openly. You might be surprised at how your story resonates with someone else and provides the encouragement they need. Similarly, offering support and encouragement to others can be incredibly rewarding. It fosters a cycle of positivity where everyone benefits from mutual encouragement. Engaging actively in discussions or leading community initiatives can enhance your commitment to your goals while helping others reach theirs, making you feel connected and understood.

Consider the story of Marty, who joined a local support group after dealing with persistent digestive issues. Initially shy, he was hesitant to share his experiences but soon found the group to be a wealth of knowledge. Members exchanged tips on everything from meal planning to stress-reduction techniques. Marty received valuable advice and supported new members, drawing from his experiences—this sense of accountability and belonging motivated him to stick to his gut-health plan despite his setbacks. Over months, Marty noticed significant improvements in his gut health and overall well-being, attributing much of his success to the supportive network he had become a part of.

Such stories highlight the impact a community can have on individual health journeys. By surrounding yourself with like-minded people, you gain access to collective knowledge and find accountability partners to help keep you on track. Whether you engage online or in person, the key is to participate actively and authentically. Share your highs and lows, ask questions, and celebrate the small victories together. In these shared moments, the true power of community is realized, helping each member move closer to their health goals.

CONTINUOUS LEARNING: STAYING INFORMED ABOUT GUT HEALTH

In the ever-evolving field of gut health, staying informed is not just beneficial—it is vital. Gut science is dynamic, with discoveries and insights emerging regularly. This makes continuous learning an essential tool for anyone looking to maintain or improve their gut health. You might wonder why keeping up with the latest research is so important. As we expand our understanding of the gut microbiome, we uncover previously unknown connections, offering new pathways to enhance wellness. These insights can lead to improved dietary choices, better management of digestive issues, and even new ways to boost mental health. By staying up-to-date, you empower yourself with the knowledge to make the best decisions about your health.

Knowing where to find reliable information is essential to keep abreast of the latest in gut health. Books and articles by reputable health experts are a great starting point. They often break down complex research into digestible insights you can apply daily. Though more technical, scientific journals provide access to cutting-edge studies and findings. If flipping through journal pages feels daunting, consider health podcasts. These often feature interviews with researchers and health professionals, offering a more casual way to absorb new information. Regarding books, look for knowledgeable authors with a knack for explaining things clearly. This ensures you are informed and understand how to apply these insights practically.

Now, with a flood of information at your fingertips, how do you discern credible sources from unreliable ones? This is where critical evaluation comes into play. Always check if the information is evidence-based and backed by expert opinions. Scientific research should be the foundation of any health advice, so look for studies and data supporting the claims. Be wary of sources that make sensationalist claims without backing them up. If something sounds too good to be true, it probably is. Beware of unverified allegations that promise miraculous results. A good rule of thumb is to cross-check information across multiple reputable sources. This practice not only reinforces the reliability of the information but also broadens your understanding by offering different perspectives.

Consider the story of Louisa, a reader who decided to dive

deeper into gut health research. Initially, she struggled with random digestive issues and low energy levels. By immersing herself in books and articles, she discovered the impact of fiber-rich diets on gut health. This prompted her to incorporate more whole grains and vegetables into her meals gradually. Over the year, she did not just see improvements in her digestion; she also felt more energetic and focused. Louisa's story highlights the transformative power of continuous learning. She could adapt her diet based on new research findings by staying informed, ultimately enhancing her well-being. Her experience is a testament to the benefits of being proactive about learning and applying new knowledge.

Staying informed is a journey filled with curiosity and discovery. As you explore the world of gut health, remember that each new insight can enhance your understanding and lifestyle. Embrace the challenge of learning, and let your curiosity guide you toward better health. Whether you read an article on the latest probiotic research or listen to a podcast about gut-brain communication, each piece of information can be a stepping stone to a healthier you.

CELEBRATING MILESTONES: ACKNOWLEDGING YOUR PROGRESS

Imagine standing at the top of a hill, looking back at the path you have climbed. Each step represents a choice, a small victory in pursuing better gut health. Recognizing your achievements along the way is not just a nice bonus—it is a powerful tool that can boost your motivation and reinforce healthy habits. Celebrating successes, no matter how small, has profound psychological benefits. It helps build confidence and self-efficacy, reinforcing the belief that you can establish and achieve goals. When you take a moment to acknowledge your progress, you are not just recognizing a single accomplishment but cultivating a mindset that values growth and perseverance. This mindset becomes a sturdy foundation that supports future achievements.

As you reach a milestone in your gut health journey, consider creative and meaningful ways to celebrate. Hosting a dinner party featuring gut-friendly recipes can be a delightful way to share your progress with loved ones. Imagine gathering friends around a table, serving dishes with flavor and nutrients while sharing stories of your health journey. Not only does this celebration highlight your achievements, but it also inspires others to explore their paths to health. Alternatively, treating yourself to a wellness activity or spa day can be a rejuvenating reward. Whether it is a relaxing massage, a manicure, a steam, or a peaceful walk in the park, these moments of self-care reinforce your commitment to well-being, offering a chance to reflect on how far you have come.

Once you have celebrated a milestone, set your sights on new goals. This practice maintains momentum and keeps your journey dynamic and engaging. Reflect on past achievements to inspire future ambitions. What have you learned about your body and health needs? How can you apply these insights to set new, challenging goals? Incremental goal setting can be particularly effective. Instead of one massive objective, break it down into smaller, manageable steps. This approach makes progress more attainable and provides frequent opportunities to celebrate. Each small success becomes a building block, gradually leading you toward your larger health aspirations.

Consider the story of Emma, who decided to reward herself with a health-focused retreat after achieving her goal of reducing her sugar intake. Initially, she struggled with constant cravings and energy slumps. However, with determination and creativity, Emma gradually incorporated more whole foods and reduced her sugar consumption. She recognized her progress and booked a weekend retreat focused on mindfulness and nutrition. The experience celebrated her achievement and provided new insights and motivation for future goals. Emma returned home refreshed and inspired, with a renewed commitment to her health journey. Her story illustrates how celebrating milestones can enhance personal growth and well-being.

The path to gut health is filled with challenges and triumphs. Acknowledging your progress and celebrating milestones reinforces the habits and mindset that drive success. Each celebration reminds you of your capabilities and resilience, encouraging you to continue exploring new possibilities for your health. As you celebrate, remember that the journey is as important as the destination. Embrace the process, learn from each experience, and savor the rewards of your efforts. In doing so, you will find that the journey to gut health is about reaching goals and enjoying the path you take to get there.

As we wrap up this chapter, remember that celebrating

milestones is integral to maintaining motivation and reinforcing healthy habits. Each celebration is a testament to your commitment and progress, serving as a stepping stone to future success. Acknowledging your achievements and setting new goals creates a dynamic and engaging journey to better gut health. With each step, you move closer to the well-being you aspire to achieve.

CONCLUSION

C ongratulations on your remarkable progress in grasping the intricate world of gut health! You have come a long way in comprehending how your gut can impact your overall well-being. Let us take a moment to review the key points we have explored. Throughout this book, we have dived into the fundamentals of the microbiome, revealing the pivotal role these trillions of microorganisms play in digestion, immunity, and mood regulation. We have emphasized the significance of probiotics, prebiotics, your gut's allies, and how they contribute to a balanced ecosystem. You have also gained insights into the fascinating gut-brain connection and how your mental health is intricately linked to your digestive system.

One of the biggest takeaways is the immense effect that gut health has on your overall wellness. Integrating gut-friendly habits into your daily routine can boost energy, balance weight, and improve mental clarity. Mindfulness and stress management are also vital, as they help maintain a healthy gut-brain axis, reducing the risk of gut-related issues. Remember, small changes can make a gigantic difference. Whether adding more fiber to your diet, practicing mindful eating, or being more aware of your body's signals, each step contributes to better health.

However, this is just the beginning. The gut-health field continuously evolves, and there is always more to discover. Please stay curious and keep exploring this fascinating subject. Engage with health communities, delve into ongoing research, and do not hesitate to seek professional counsel when necessary. The more you learn, the better equipped you will be to make informed health decisions.

Now, it is time to take action. Take what you have learned and start applying these strategies to your life. Keep a gut-health journal to track your progress and identify what works best for you. Share your experiences with others—friends or online communities—to build support and accountability. The journey to a healthier gut is personal, but you are not alone. Together, we can make a community that encourages and inspires each other.

I want to acknowledge your dedication to reading this book. By doing so, you have taken a proactive step toward better health, which is something to be proud of. Every small change you make counts, and your efforts bring you closer to your wellness goals. Your journey is unique, and any progress is a victory, no matter how small. You are on the right track.

Thank you for choosing this book as your guide. I appreciate your trust and engagement, and I sincerely hope the information shared here will be valuable in your pursuit of a healthier lifestyle. If you have questions or need further guidance, remember that resources are available. Look for online platforms, newsletters, and social media channels where you can continue learning and connecting with others interested in gut health.

As we wrap up, I want to leave you an inspirational note. The path to better health does not have to be overwhelming. It is about making small, consistent efforts that lead to significant improvements over time. Embrace this journey with optimism and determination, knowing each positive choice contributes to lasting wellness. Your gut health is just one aspect of your overall well-being, but it is powerful. With every step, you empower yourself to live a healthier, more fulfilling life. Here is to your continued success and vibrant health!

APPENDIX: GUT HEALTH ACROSS OUR LIFESPANS

Understanding that our gut microbiome is not a fixed entity but rather an evolving system influenced by various factors at each stage of life is crucial. From birth to our golden years, gut health is a cornerstone of our overall well-being, adapting to different life phases and challenges. This knowledge galvanizes us to make educated choices about supporting our gut health, regardless of age. This chapter delves into the evolution of gut health and provides specific strategies for each stage, equipping you with the tools to take charge of your gut health journey.

CHILDHOOD AND GUT DEVELOPMENT

The foundation of lifelong gut health is laid in early childhood, with the first three years being particularly crucial for microbiome development. During birth, babies receive their first exposure to beneficial bacteria, either through vaginal delivery or cesarean section. This initial colonization sets the stage for future gut health. However, breastfeeding further enriches the infant microbiome, providing essential prebiotics through human milk oligosaccharides and protective antibodies that support immune system development, making it a key factor in the early development of gut health.

As children transition to solid foods, their gut microbiome undergoes significant changes. This period represents a critical window for establishing healthy eating habits and a diverse microbiome. Exposure to whole foods, mainly fruits, vegetables, and fiber-rich foods, is crucial during this phase as it helps cultivate a robust and diverse gut ecosystem. Common childhood challenges like picky eating or frequent antibiotic use can impact this development, making implementing strategies that support healthy gut colonization essential.

The preschool and early school years bring new challenges and opportunities for gut health. Exposure to different environments, including daycare and school settings, continues to shape the developing microbiome. During this time, supporting immune function through gut health becomes particularly important as children encounter various pathogens and develop resistance to common illnesses. Establishing routines around healthy eating, regular mealtimes, and proper hygiene helps create a foundation for lifelong gut health.

ADOLESCENT GUT HEALTH

Adolescence dramatically changes body chemistry and lifestyle habits, significantly impacting gut health. Hormonal fluctuations during puberty can affect digestive function and the composition of gut bacteria. These changes often coincide with increased independence in food choices, potentially leading to dietary patterns that may not support optimal gut health. The stress of academic pressures, social relationships, and other teenage challenges can also influence digestive wellness through the gut-brain axis.

During this period, teenagers often experiment with different diets, sometimes adopting restrictive eating patterns that can compromise gut health. The increased autonomy in food choices might lead to higher consumption of these foods and irregular eating schedules. Additionally, changes in sleep patterns and increased exposure to environmental factors like stress and peer pressure can affect the sensitive balance of gut bacteria.

Supporting adolescent gut health requires a balanced approach that acknowledges biological and lifestyle changes. Education about the connection between diet, mood, and gut health becomes crucial during this time. Encouraging healthy food choices while maintaining flexibility helps teenagers develop a positive relationship with food that supports their growing bodies and changing nutritional needs. As a teenager, you may face numerous challenges, but understanding the importance of a healthy diet and its impact on your gut health can make you feel supported and understood in your journey toward adulthood.

PREGNANCY AND POSTPARTUM

Pregnancy initiates a cascade of changes in the gut microbiome that affect both the mother and the developing baby. Hormonal changes during pregnancy alter digestive function and bacterial composition, sometimes leading to common issues like morning sickness and constipation. The maternal microbiome is essential in fetal development, influencing everything from immune system development to potential disease risk in the child.

The dramatic hormonal shifts of pregnancy can challenge digestive comfort, but they serve important purposes in preparing for birth and lactation. Supporting gut health during pregnancy becomes particularly important as the maternal microbiome influences the baby's initial bacterial colonization. Specific dietary considerations during this time include adequate fiber intake, probiotic-rich foods, and proper hydration to support maternal and fetal health.

The postpartum period brings its own set of challenges for gut health. Recovery from birth, hormonal fluctuations, and the demands of caring for a newborn can impact digestive function. For breastfeeding mothers, maintaining optimal gut health becomes even more crucial as it can affect milk production and composition. This period requires particular attention to nutrient-dense foods that support healing and recovery while maintaining digestive comfort.

AGING AND THE MICROBIOME

As we age, our gut microbiome naturally undergoes significant changes that can impact our overall health and well-being. Reduced digestive enzyme production, changes in stomach acid levels, and slower gut motility can all affect how we process and absorb nutrients. Understanding these age-related changes helps us develop strategies to maintain optimal gut function throughout our later years.

The aging gut faces several challenges, including reduced microbial diversity, increased inflammation, and decreased immune function. These changes can contribute to common age-related health concerns and impact quality of life. Factors such as medication use, particularly antibiotics and acid reducers, can further affect the delicate balance of gut bacteria. Additionally, changes in appetite and eating habits may lead to reduced intake of fiber and other nutrients essential for gut health.

Supporting the aging microbiome requires targeted strategies that address these specific challenges. Maintaining regular physical activity, ensuring adequate fiber intake, and including fermented foods can help preserve microbial diversity. Special attention to hydration becomes crucial, as older adults often have a lowered sense of thirst. Regular probiotic supplementation might be beneficial, particularly after courses of antibiotics or during increased susceptibility to infections.

The key to maintaining gut health throughout aging is adapting strategies to changing needs while maintaining consistency in core healthy habits. These include regular meal times, adequate hydration, and attention to fiber intake. Social connections around meals and maintaining the pleasure of eating also support gut health and overall well-being in later years.

Bibliography

Defining the Human Microbiome, https://pmc.ncbi.nlm.nih.gov/articles/PMC3426293/

Benefits of Probiotic Foods: Using good bacteria for better health, https://www.health.harvard.edu/digestive-health/benefits-of-probiotic-foods-using-good-bacteria-for-better-health

What are probiotics and prebiotics? https://www.mayoclinic.org/healthy-lifestyle/nutrition-and-healthy-eating/expert-answers/probiotics/faq-20058065

The gut-brain axis: interactions between enteric microbiota, central and enteric nervous systems, https://pmc.ncbi.nlm.nih.gov/articles/PMC4367209/

Diversity, stability and resilience of the human gut microbiota, https://pmc.ncbi.nlm.nih.gov/articles/PMC3577372/

Dietary Fibre Modulates the Gut Microbiota, https://pmc.ncbi.nlm.nih.gov/articles/PMC8153313/

Leaky gut: What is it, and what does it mean for you? https://www.health.harvard.edu/blog/leaky-gut-what-is-it-and-what-does-it-mean-for-you-2017092212451

Research says gut-brain axis plays role in mental health, https://www.uclahealth.org/news/article/research-says-gut-brain-axis-plays-role-mental-health

Gut-Skin Axis: Unravelling the Connection between the Gut Microbiome and Psoriasis, https://pubmed.ncbi.nlm.nih.gov/35625774/

What to know about SIBO and its treatment, https://www.medicalnewstoday.com/articles/324475

Exploring the Influence of Gut Microbiome on Energy Metabolism in Humans, https://pmc.ncbi.nlm.nih.gov/articles/PMC10334151/

Role of the Gut Microbiome in Weight Management, https://tristategastro.net/role-of-the-gut-microbiome-in-weight-management/

Mindful Eating: A Review Of How The Stress-Digestion-Mindfulness Triad May Modulate And Improve Gastrointestinal And Digestive Function, https://pmc.ncbi.nlm.nih.gov/articles/PMC7219460/

Stress Reduction for Irritable Bowel Syndrome, https://nyulangone.org/conditions/irritable-bowel-syndrome/treatments/stress-reduction-for-irritable-bowel-syndrome

Best Gut Health Apps of 2020, https://www.healthline.com/health/digestive-health/top-iphone-android-apps-gut-health

30 recipes for a healthy gut, https://www.olivemagazine.com/recipes/collection/recipes-healthy-gut/

The Benefits of Whole Foods: How a Holistic Diet Can Boost Your Energy and Immune System, https://modernnutritionandpilates.com/blogupdates/2023/9/13/the-benefits-of-whole-foods-how-a-holistic-diet-can-boost-your-energy-and-immune-system

How to get more probiotics, https://www.health.harvard.edu/staying-healthy/how-to-get-more-probiotics

The Top Foods to Avoid for a Healthy Gut, https://www.gastroconsa.com/the-top-foods-to-avoid-for-a-healthy-gut/

Does drinking water during or after a meal affect or disturb digestion? https://www.mayoclinic.org/healthy-lifestyle/nutrition-and-healthy-eating/expert-answers/digestion/faq-20058348

Factors Determining Effective Probiotic Activity: Evaluation of Survival and Antibacterial Activity of Selected Probiotic Products Using an "In Vitro" Study, https://pmc.ncbi.nlm.nih.gov/articles/PMC9413312/

What are probiotics and prebiotics? https://www.mayoclinic.org/healthy-lifestyle/nutrition-and-healthy-eating/expert-answers/probiotics/faq-20058065

6 Conscious Probiotic Supplement Brands for a Healthy Gut, https://www.considerbeyond.com/lets-consider-beyond/optimizing-womens-well-being-top-3-supplements-for-daily-gut-health-harmony

The Ultimate Meal Prepping Guide For Busy Schedules, https://fitonapp.com/nutrition/meal-planning-with-a-busy-schedule/

How to eat healthy in social settings: 9 tips for staying on track, https://www.noom.com/blog/nutrition/how-to-eat-healthy-in-social-settings-9-tips-for-staying-on-track/

Stress, depression, diet, and the gut microbiota: human–bacteria interactions at the core of psychoneuroimmunology and nutrition, https://pmc.ncbi.nlm.nih.gov/articles/PMC7213601/

Probiotic Myths, https://www.optibacprobiotics.com/learning-lab/probiotic-myths

The Gut-Brain Axis: Influence of Microbiota on Mood and Mental Health, https://pmc.ncbi.nlm.nih.gov/articles/PMC6469458/

The gut-brain connection, https://www.health.harvard.edu/diseases-and-conditions/the-gut-brain-connection

BIBLIOGRAPHY

Gut Health: How Deep Meditation Can Improve It, https://www.healthline.com/health-news/gut-health-how-deep-meditation-can-improve-it

The Poop About Your Gut Health and Personalized Nutrition, https://www.wired.com/story/gut-health-personalized-nutrition/

How Journaling Can Improve Your Gut Health, https://www.dr-gupta.com/post/how-journaling-can-improve-your-gut-health

Exploring the gut microbiota: lifestyle choices, disease associations, and personal genomics, https://www.frontiersin.org/journals/nutrition/articles/10.3389/fnut.2023.1225120/full

What to Look for in a Gut Health Nutritionist, https://www.topnutritioncoaching.com/blog/what-to-look-for-in-a-gut-health-nutritionist

Simple Lifestyle Changes for Better Gut Health, https://integrishealth.org/resources/on-your-health/2023/october/simple-lifestyle-changes-for-better-gut-health

Gut microbes are the community within you that you can't live without – how eating well can cultivate your microbial and social self, https://theconversation.com/gut-microbes-are-the-community-within-you-that-you-cant-live-without-how-eating-well-can-cultivate-your-microbial-and-social-self-210668

Gut microbiome in 2023: current and emerging research trends, https://www.gutmicrobiotaforhealth.com/gut-microbiome-in-2023-current-and-emerging-research-trends/

www.ingramcontent.com/pod-product-compliance
Lightning Source LLC
Chambersburg PA
CBHW071233210326
41597CB00016B/2037